Getting Research Published

An A to Z of publication strategy

Second Edition

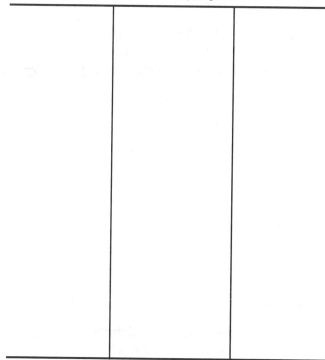

Radcliffe Publishing Ltd
18 Marcham Road
Abingdon
Oxon OX14 1AA
United Kingdom

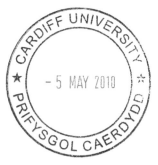

www.radcliffe-oxford.com
Electronic catalogue and worldwide online ordering facility.

First Edition 2005

British Library Cataloguing in Publication Data

A catalogue record for this book is available from the British Library.

ISBN-13: 978 184619 408 5

The paper used for the text pages of this book
is FSC certified. FSC (The Forest Stewardship
Council) is an international network to promote
responsible management of the world's forests.

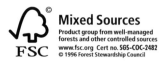

Mixed Sources
Product group from well-managed
forests and other controlled sources
www.fsc.org Cert no. SGS-COC-2482
© 1996 Forest Stewardship Council

FSC

Typeset by Pindar New Zealand, Auckland, New Zealand
Printed and bound by TJI Digital, Padstow, Cornwall, UK

Contents

Foreword to second edition

Getting published is extremely important for a great many people. Promotion, grants, distinction, riches, and, as Freud put it in a more sexist age, 'fame and the love of beautiful women' can all flow from publication.

But there are also strong, less selfish reasons for publishing. We in rich countries overwhelmed with published material may forget that writing, publishing, critically reading, and debating are fundamental to any system that wants to improve – and certainly for any health system.

I'm writing this on a plane returning from Nigeria, and sadly Nigeria's health system might not unkindly be described as failed.

Joseph Ana, a friend of mine and the editor of *BMJ West Africa*, took over as health commissioner in Cross River State, one of the poorest states in Nigeria, five years ago, and after visiting every part of the region documented the dire state of the health system. It was failing at every level but especially at the primary care level where facilities were dilapidated and services barely functioning. People had no confidence in the system and went elsewhere to get care and give birth. Maternal mortality was 1%, childhood mortality 20%, and immunisation rates under 20%; and there were only 72 doctors for 3 million people.

Enhanced information flow will, Joseph believes, play an essential part in improving the health system. Indeed, a flow of good information and vigorous debate are in themselves an essential part of a well functioning health system.

So there are very strong and unselfish reasons for publishing, but old lags like me, who have published and been rejected all over the place and roundly abused for some of the nonsense we've written, underestimate how terrifying and difficult it can be to get started in the publishing game.

This is where Liz Wager's book is so helpful. It provides a very readable and authoritative guide to every aspect of publishing in scientific journals, and the book's layout means that readers are both provided with a route map for publishing but can also find quickly information on the topics that might be bothering them. Perhaps the greatest tribute I can pay to the book is that I shamefully lifted some of the material for the workshop on publishing that I was running in Nigeria. The audience found the information extremely useful, and I thoroughly recommended the book to them – as I do to you.

Richard Smith
Former editor, *BMJ*
Director, UnitedHealth Chronic Disease Initiative
January 2010

Foreword to first edition

Contemporary biomedical research has turned one traditional image of the scientist – the isolated figure, toiling alone, in a small, cluttered, dimly lit laboratory, late at night – into a quaint anachronism. The scale and complexity of today's research projects usually require large teams of people, who may be scattered across the world, with highly specialised skills. Despite the teamwork now inherent in most research, one part of the process, writing up the resulting paper, remains essentially a solitary undertaking.

This approach is curious indeed. Why venture into the wilds without a guide? Who thinks it's a good idea to light out for unknown territory without a map? Would you hand a scalpel to a novice and send him into the operating theatre alone? Of course not. This is, however, just the sort of experience plenty of junior researchers have once the trial is over, the experiments are done, and the data have been analysed: they receive the earnest but empty directive to 'go write it up'. And here they may be following in the footsteps of their seniors, who probably navigated the publications process in a similar trial-and-error manner – doubtless heavier on the latter than on the former.

At last, help is at hand. *Getting Research Published: An A to Z of publication strategy* is a kind of guide to the perplexed. It will be useful to those who recognise they're perplexed by the process of writing and publishing, and helpful even to those who don't know what they don't know. (I even venture to suggest that we editors might learn a thing or two from it.) In this volume, Liz Wager provides just the sort of lively and intelligent guidance that will be warmly received by everyone who wants to publish research results. The format is user-friendly, the advice up to date, sound and tempered by pragmatism. Wager wears her considerable learning lightly, with a judicious selection of references and resources. Her recommendations are evidence-based where possible, and qualified accordingly when evidence is lacking. As an active researcher, writer, teacher and advocate, she is highly qualified to synthesise and assess the literature of publishing research. Last, but hardly least, her enthusiasm and sense of humour are evident and most welcome.

Carrying out scientific research and seeing it into print are never going to be easy tasks. But by arming themselves with this guide, researchers can assure themselves of a better informed, easier and altogether more pleasant path to publication.

Faith McLellan
former North American Senior Editor, *The Lancet*
President, Council of Science Editors
March 2005

About this book

This book has been written for everybody involved with getting biomedical and healthcare research published. Most of the book follows an A to Z format. I decided to arrange the information in this way because every publication poses different problems. I also hoped that this style would make the information relevant and accessible to readers with varying levels of experience and from different backgrounds, including individuals writing up their own research and people coordinating complex publication projects for research funders.

However, one problem with an A to Z format is that you need to have some idea of what to look for and it is not helpful for times when you don't know what you don't know. I have therefore included an overview at the beginning which contains a few longer sections to set the scene. If you are new to publications, I suggest you read the overview first and, if any terms are unfamiliar or any parts do not make sense, start diving into the rest of the book. Throughout the book, terms that appear in the A to Z are shown in **bold**.

I have not used references in the academic manner to support every statement but have included suggestions for further reading or useful websites within entries where this seemed helpful. Although some of the conventions of peer review date back to the 18th century, other aspects are evolving rapidly and, since starting to write the first edition in mid-2004, and updating it in 2009, there have been several important developments affecting publications. I therefore urge readers to get into the habit of scanning major journals and keeping an eye on relevant websites (e.g. www.thepublicationplan.com) to stay up to date.

One reason for writing this book is that information about publishing research is scattered and some conventions seem never to have been written down. Many journal instructions to authors seem to hark back to a time when one or two collaborators wrote up their own, small research projects and do not reflect the realities of large-scale multicentre trials. Another reason is that journals and meetings do not all function in a uniform way. With over 20 000 medical journals in existence you would not be able to lift a volume that covered every requirement of every title, even if it had been possible to compile such a mammoth text. Many of the statements in this book are therefore generalisations. I have tried to guide readers around likely problems and offer solutions based on my experiences gathered over 20 years of writing, editing and coordinating publications for drug companies and individual researchers. I hope you find it helpful, but please remember to check the requirements of individual journals and meetings before assuming that I am right.

Elizabeth Wager
January 2010

About the author

Liz Wager is a freelance publications consultant, trainer, writer and editor. She has worked with doctors, drug companies, journal editors and writers on five continents. She studied zoology at Oxford and Reading but discovered she was better at writing about research than doing it. Before setting up her own company, Sideview, she worked for Blackwell Scientific Publications as an editor, was the medical writer for Janssen-Cilag in the UK, and then UK head of international medical publications at Glaxo Wellcome. Working in the pharmaceutical industry she developed an interest in publication ethics and led a group that published Good Publication Practice for Pharmaceutical Companies. She currently chairs COPE (the Committee on Publication Ethics) and is a member of the ethics committees of the BMJ and the World Association of Medical Editors. She has done research into peer review (which, unlike zoology, does not involve operating temperamental equipment or washing-up) including Cochrane reviews on the effects of peer review and technical editing. She has written articles and book chapters on various aspects of scientific publishing and is a co-author of *How to Survive Peer Review* (BMJ Books, 2002). She is a Visiting Fellow of the UK Cochrane Centre. She lives in Buckinghamshire with her long-suffering husband and three tortoiseshell cats (who have to put up with her habit of reading medical journals in bed).

Sideview
Princes Risborough
E-mail: liz@sideview.demon.co.uk

Part One

Publication Strategy – an Overview

CHAPTER 1

Step-by-step guide to publication strategy

Most of this book does not follow a step-by-step approach because each publication will raise fresh issues and readers have different needs. If you already have questions or problems I suggest you use the A to Z section to find the information you need, but if you want a general overview the following steps are designed to help you navigate around the book and reflect the stages common to most research publications. **Bold** print indicates an entry in the A to Z section, which you should consult if you do not understand the term or want more detail.

1 *Identify the key message.* (What do you want the publication to say?) For example, your findings show that Tumorzap increases life expectancy in patients with advanced cancer. That is your **key message**. Remember that a message needs a verb (i.e. an action word, in this case 'increases'). A statement, without a verb, such as 'The efficacy of Tumorzap in advanced cancer', is not a message.

2 *Identify the **target audience(s).*** (Who might be interested in your message?) The primary audience for this study would be oncologists, with a secondary audience of haematologists.

3 *Finalise the authors and **writing group** for this publication.* Ideally, you will have agreed some ground rules for **authorship** at the start of the study. The writing group may also include a professional writer who is not an author.

4 *Agree responsibilities for preparing and reviewing the publication.* Remember that a wider group of people than just the authors will probably need to review the publication. This may include sign-off from the research sponsor or approval from a head of department.

5 *Agree the **target journal** and a **second target** in case your paper is rejected by the first.* See **journal choice** for more details.

6 *Agree a timetable and a list of responsibilities.* (Who will do what?) Send these to all the **key people**.

7 *Prepare an **outline**.* This is especially helpful if several people are drafting different sections or if the paper is being prepared by a professional writer who is not an author. All authors should get a chance to comment on the outline. This will save time and avoid disagreements later.

8 *Prepare the first draft.* There are plenty of books about **writing** but most start from this stage. For successful, and pain-free, publishing, you also need to pay attention to steps 1 to 7.

9 *At the same time:*

- gather authors' comments, circulate them and prepare subsequent drafts. This process continues until you reach consensus. While you might feel exhilarated and excited when you prepare the first draft, you will almost certainly experience other times when you feel fed up, frustrated and demotivated. Resolving petty disagreements between **co-authors** and doing tedious jobs like organising references are never much fun, but keep your publication goal in mind. Although word processing and e-mail have revolutionised the process of circulating drafts, collating comments and redrafting papers, the disadvantage of electronic communication is that you may rarely speak to, let alone actually see, your co-authors. Picking up the telephone or having a face-to-face meeting may lift your spirits and renew your energy. It is also often the quickest way to resolve minor differences over wording and definitely preferable to endless e-mail 'ping-pong'. If at all possible, plan at least two **meetings** of the writing group: the first to discuss the data and agree the overall strategy (key message, target audience, etc.), the second to agree the final draft just before submission.
- consult (**internal review**). This goes on in parallel with the tasks in the bullet point above. Who you need to consult depends on the nature of the research and how it was organised and funded. It also depends on the skills of the author(s) and writing group. Consider showing drafts to the following people.

Table 1.1: Internal reviewers

Reviewer	Focus of review
Statistician	Data presentation, statistics
Senior colleague	Methodology, presentation, journal preferences
Native English speaker	Language
Practising clinician not involved in research	Practical implications, discussion
Librarian/Information scientist	References
Naïve reader (partner, parent, friend)	Logical flow
Nitpicker	Annoying mistakes

10 *Prepare the submission package.* Draft the **covering letter** and make sure you have gathered everything you need for submission. This might include (depending on the journal):

- **copyright** transfer form
- signed declarations of **authorship**
- signed statements from everyone listed in the **acknowledgements** section
- statements on **competing interest**
- **permissions** to reproduce figures.

Check the title page for: author **names**, qualifications, **affiliations**, full contact details for **corresponding author**, details of individual contributions. Re-check the journal's instructions for other bits and pieces you might have forgotten such as: **key words, running title**, word count.

Check the journal's requirements for things like page numbering, justification (e.g. ragged right-hand text edge) and page breaks. These are especially important if you submit a paper electronically.

11 *Submit the paper.* But only after everybody is happy with it . . . and don't forget to let the key people know that the paper has been submitted.

12 *Wait patiently.* Or start work on your next publication.

13 *(unlucky for some . . .) The decision.* Inform everybody as soon as you get a decision. If it is a rejection, consider the reviewers' comments and revise the paper if they have identified remediable problems or simple mistakes, but do not waste time feeling dejected. Get agreement on any revisions and submit to the second **target journal** as soon as possible.

If you get a **conditional acceptance**, discuss the reviewers' comments with all authors and agree a response. Revise the manuscript and make a list of the changes you have made. Agree the revisions, then resubmit.

14 *Acceptance.* At last, all that work has paid off. You can now quote the paper as being 'in press'.

15 *Wait patiently (again).* How long you have to wait will depend a great deal on your **journal choice**. The period between acceptance and publication is known as the **lead time**. Use it constructively to agree how many **offprints** to order (*see* step 17).

16 *Check proofs.* These will be sent to the **corresponding author**.

17 *Order offprints.* An offprint form is often sent out with the proofs and will need to be returned without delay. To save time, find out how much offprints cost and agree how many everybody wants as soon as the paper has been accepted. Offprints ordered at the time of publication are usually cheaper than **reprints** ordered later.

18 *Publication.* Relish the moment! Your strategy has been successful. Bask in the glory and recommend this book to somebody else if it has been helpful!

19 *Follow-up.* Be prepared to respond to correspondence published in the journal. If readers (or you) spot a mistake, contact the editor to discuss publishing a **correction (erratum)**. Send out **reprints** or electronic copies to people who request them.

20 *Evaluate.* Learn from your successes, failures and mistakes. Even a rejection or a tedious wait gives you information about what to do next time. If you are licking your wounds from a particularly unpleasant dispute about authorship or smarting from torrents of abuse from a disgruntled author (or editor), think about what you might have done differently to prevent these situations from arising. If you are handling a lot of publications, keep notes of **journal decision times** and **lead times**. These will build up into a useful resource for the next time you choose a target journal.

CHAPTER 2

Developing a publication plan for a multicentre study

Ideally, publication plans should be developed at the earliest stages of trial planning. Thinking about potential publications as you design the protocol can increase your chances of producing publishable results. Early planning and clear communication can also prevent later problems with authorship.

For large, multicentre studies, it is unfeasible for all investigators to be named as authors on publications. It is therefore helpful to agree **authorship** criteria at the start of the study. This will avoid many problems caused by unrealistic **expectations** or misunderstandings. At the outset, it may not be possible to predict exactly who will qualify as authors, but it is usually possible to agree how authorship will be allotted. The protocol development team (which usually comprises clinicians or senior scientists from the sponsor, a statistician and three or four key investigators) is a good starting point for a **writing group**, but, in the course of the study, personnel may change, so you cannot necessarily predict the exact composition of the final group, nor exactly who will qualify as authors.

Ground rules for invitation to join a writing team might be:

- protocol development team plus one investigator from each centre (to be nominated by each centre), or
- principal investigator, statistician, plus top recruiting investigator from each country, or
- principal investigator, five top recruiting investigators, plus company employees who meet ICMJE criteria.

Authors' responsibilities should be discussed and agreed at the outset. An invitation to join a writing team should not be viewed as an automatic qualification for authorship. Authors must expect to contribute to data interpretation and developing the publication.

Ground rules for authorship should be clearly communicated to everybody involved with the study, so that disagreements can be resolved promptly, and everybody has the same expectations.

Some companies and, to a lesser extent, academic institutions have their own authorship policies. These may be helpful (you should certainly be aware of them) but, if you consider the policy contravenes journal authorship criteria, such as the **International Committee of Medical Journal Editors (ICMJE)** criteria, you should be prepared to challenge them.

Authorship policies that may fall foul of accepted criteria include:

- never permitting employees to be named as authors on papers relating to company products
- only permitting a set number of employees to be named as authors (e.g. one per paper)
- always requiring an employee or particular individual (e.g. head of department, or professor) to be included as an author.

Such policies are likely to create problems of **ghost** or **guest authors**. It is much better to agree ground rules for each study.

Thinking about publications can also help to focus the study design. Imagining how the results might appear in a journal may help to identify weaknesses and omissions. Involving patients or carers in clinical trial design is good practice, and may also help to identify interesting publications or increase the scope of potential publications, e.g. by including a quality of life assessment.

Publication strategies (and especially plans for authorship) should be clearly set out and communicated, preferably in writing within the **investigators' agreement** or as a separate **publication agreement**.

Identifying target meetings can help to plan study timing – although this inevitably involves some crystal ball gazing, so you should not expect to be too precise. However, aiming to submit an abstract by a certain deadline may help to focus minds. If you wait to create your strategy until the data are ready, you might find you have needlessly missed a crucial deadline by a few days. Thinking about likely publications may also help to develop the **data analysis plan**, e.g. by identifying sub-group analyses at the outset.

An example of an outline publication strategy at the start of a study is shown in Table 2.1.

Once the results are available, the plan can be refined. At this stage, you should identify the authors, **key messages** and target meeting/journal for each publication. An example is given in Table 2.2.

You should also produce a detailed timetable and circulate it to everybody who will be involved with the publication. Agreeing a timetable is particularly crucial if you have tight deadlines to meet. It also helps by setting out the steps to publication. These vary, depending on the complexity of the publication (which will affect how many drafts and review rounds you might need) and the study sponsor/organisers (who will have different requirements for review and approval).

If several people, or several organisations, are involved in developing a publication, a detailed plan can also be helpful in identifying who is responsible for each action or stage. A possible plan is shown in Table 2.3.

Table 2.1: Outline publication strategy prepared at the start of a study

Publication	Topic	Meeting/Journal	Target audience	Submission deadline/target	Publication date
Abstract 1	Efficacy data	ESMO	Oncologists	May 10	Nov. 10
Abstract 2	Safety data	ESMO	Oncologists	May 10	Nov. 10
Abstract 3	Sub-group data (haem)	EHA	Haematologists	Jan. 11	June 11
Abstract 4	Quality of life	*Cancer Nursing*	Oncology nurses	Feb. 11	Aug. 11
Main paper	Main results	Oncology (?JCO)	Oncologists	Q3 10	Q1 11
Paper 2	Sub-group analyses	Haematology (?Blood)	Haematologists	Q1 11	Q3 11
Paper 3	Long-term follow-up	Oncology	Oncologists	2012	?

(Q = quarter; thus Q3 10 indicates the third quarter of 2010)

Table 2.2: More detailed plan prepared when results are available

Publication	Key message	Authors	Meeting/ Journal
Abstract 1	Tumorzap increases survival in cancer patients	X, Y, Z	ESMO
Abstract 2	Tumorzap causes less nausea than Chemowiz	Y, Z, X	ESMO
Abstract 3	Tumorzap induces complete remission in some haematological malignancies	Z, X, H	EHA
Abstract 4	Tumorzap improves patient quality of life	X, Y, Q	*Cancer Nursing*
Main paper (P1)	Tumorzap increases survival and is well tolerated in patients with advanced cancer	X, Y, H, Q, Z	*JCO*
Paper 2	Tumorzap induces complete remission in some haematological malignancies	Z, X, H	*Blood*
Paper 3	Long-term (two-year) follow-up confirms survival benefit with Tumorzap	Y, X, Z	*Ann Onc*

Table 2.3: Detailed publication plan showing timelines and responsibilities

Publication	Data ready	1st draft	Writing group review	Collate comments write 2nd draft	Xth draft	Internal company review	All authors final review	Submit	Decision expected	Publication expected	Current status
A1	5 April (Stats)	15 April AW	30 April	5 May AW	...	10 May SM	12 May	15 May PA	July	30 Oct. 10	Submitted
P1	5 April (Stats)	5 May AW	26 May	10 June AW	...	1 July SM	10 July	17 July CA	mid-Sept.	Jan. 11	Drafted

Key: AW = a writer; SM = senior medic; PA = presenting author; CA = **corresponding author**

CHAPTER 3

How long will it take?

Converting your publication strategy into a realistic plan requires some surprising skills. If you bought this book hoping that it would have handy tables showing exactly how long everything will take, you may be disappointed. It is possible to give broad estimates, but each publication is different and the timetable will depend on all sorts of intangible things like whether the authors work well together and how much priority the **key players** give to (and therefore how much time and resources they are prepared to invest in) the publication.

However, there are two tricks to publication planning. The first is to make the plan as detailed as possible. The second is to be as pessimistic as possible. Breaking the plan into small chunks should ensure that you have not omitted any vital stages. It also means that you will quickly realise if timings slip and might be able to do something about it (or, at the very least, adjust the other timings). A recipe for disaster is a 'plan' (it hardly deserves the name) that simply states that the study data will be available in April 2011 and the primary paper will be published in September 2011. Given the right choice of journal and an extraordinarily dedicated and cooperative bunch of authors, this timing might be possible, but, to be of any use, a plan must break down the stages, otherwise you cannot tell anything is amiss until you miss your target publication date, and it is too late.

Chapter 2 'Developing a publication plan for a multicentre study' (pp. 7–11) should give you some ideas of the stages you need to include. The most obvious ones are:

- form a **writing group** and agree **key message(s), target audience** and target meeting(s)/journal
- prepare an **outline**
- get agreement on the **outline** from all **key players**
- prepare **first draft**
- circulate draft and collate comments
- consult with people outside the writing group (**informal review**)
- continue process until consensus is reached (this stage is by far the most unpredictable and can drag on for ages)
- get approval to submit (this usually involves review by sponsor and/or institution)
- prepare submission package (**covering letter, permissions,** etc.)
- submit publication
- receive decision and reviewers' comments
- either respond to comments (if you get a **conditional acceptance**) or submit to second target journal if your paper is rejected
- receive acceptance

- check **proofs** and order **offprints**
- celebrate the publication!

Surprisingly, preparing the first draft is often relatively straightforward, especially if you are working from a well-prepared protocol and statistical report. However, here are some stages that could trip you up:

- obtaining permission for reproducing **figures** and tables from other publications
- getting figures professionally drawn
- gathering all the information needed for the submission package
- internal review by the sponsor.

Did I hear a faint howl of anguish, or at least a slight muttering when I wrote that this book would not contain handy tables? The point I am trying to make is that, to be realistic, each plan must take account of all the factors affecting each individual publication and that a 'one-size-fits-all' approach (e.g. six months to publish any paper) is doomed to failure: but here are a few tables.

Table 3.1: Timing for pre-submission stages for an 'average' research paper

Stage	Best case	Average	But it could take . . .
Organise meeting, agree strategy	1 week	4 weeks	3 months
Prepare outline	1 week	2 weeks	1 month
Agree outline	1 week	2 weeks	1 month
Prepare first draft	2 weeks	4 weeks	3 months
Consult/reach consensus	4 weeks	10 weeks	4 months
Internal review/approval	2 weeks	4 weeks	3 months
Prepare submission package/ submit	1 week	2 weeks	2 months
Total	**3 months**	**7 months**	**17 months**

Table 3.2: Timing for abstracts

Stage	Speedy	Sluggish
Agree strategy	1 week	4 weeks
Prepare first draft	1 week	2 weeks
Consult/reach consensus	2 weeks	4 weeks
Internal review/approval	2 weeks	4 weeks
Submit	1 day	1 week
Total	**6 weeks +**	**15 weeks**

Table 3.3: How long do journals take?

Stage	Rapid[1]	Fast track[2]	Moderate[3]	Dinosaurs[4]
Decision – reject	2–10 days		1–3 months	3–6 months
Decision – accept	2–4 weeks	1–3 days	3–4 months	3–6 months
Allow time to respond to reviewers' comments – that's up to you!				
Final acceptance	1 week		1 month	3 months
Lead time (acceptance to publication) – web[5]	1–5 days		Variable	6–12 months
Lead time – printed version	4 weeks		3–4 months	6–12 months
Total (acceptance to publication)	**3–12 weeks**	**4 weeks**	**7–9 months**	**12–21 months**

1 Examples of rapid publications are journals such as *Current Medical Research & Opinion* or expedited review in the *International Journal of Clinical Practice*.
2 This applies to the *British Medical Journal* (*BMJ*) and *The Lancet* **fast track**.
3 Moderate – this mainly applies to weekly journals, such as the *BMJ* and *The Lancet* (regular, not fast track).
4 Dinosaurs – this applies to most specialty journals – the lower figures generally apply to monthly journals and the higher figures to less frequent (e.g. quarterly) journals, but there are exceptions.
5 Many journals publish on their website before the print version, although traditional journals tend to publish both versions at the same time. The time to web publication is not included in the total figure, because it does not affect the lead time to printing. For purely electronic journals, e.g. *PLoS Medicine*, there is no printed version, so final publication occurs on the web.

Research your target journal carefully to find out where it fits. The important message of this table is that **journal choice** is often the most important factor in determining the speed of publication.

■ How long do conferences take?

Abstracts are either rejected or accepted, there is no messing around with conditional acceptances or responding to reviewers' comments. The meeting dates are fixed, but there is considerable variation in submission deadlines.

Table 3.4: Timings for conferences

	Small/regional meeting or 'late breaker'[1]	*Major international meeting*
Time to decision	1–3 months	2–4 months
Time from acceptance to meeting	1–3 months	4–8 months
Total from submission deadline to meeting	2–6 months	4–12 months

1   Some large meetings permit **'late breaker' abstracts** – this is the equivalent of the journal fast track and is usually reserved for new and interesting data.

■ General rules

Once you have worked on several publications with a core group, you will get a feel for how long they usually take. It is much harder to estimate how long a publication will take to develop if the writing group has not worked together before. A number of factors will influence the timetable and, while you cannot usually do anything to change these, at least you can take them into account if you are trying to plan, as shown in Table 3.5.

Table 3.5: Factors affecting the time it takes to develop a publication

Factors encouraging rapid publication	*Factors that tend to slow down publication*
Small writing group (< six people)	Large writing group (≥ six people)
Writing group members can meet easily	It is difficult/costly to arrange meetings (e.g. members are widely scattered)
Writing group members know and like each other	Writing group members have not worked together before, or do not get on well
Writing and publication experience	Lack of publication experience
Stable membership of group/other players	Changing personnel throughout study and while developing publication (e.g. statisticians, writers, sponsor representatives)
Effective leadership of writing group (e.g. inspirational principal investigator)	Tension within writing group (e.g. battles for seniority or several people with strong and differing opinions)
Straightforward methods (e.g. similar design has been published before)	New design or complex study
Straightforward results (i.e. clear interpretation, everybody agrees on what they mean)	Controversial or inconclusive results/lack of agreement about interpretation
All key players give the publication high priority	Publication has low priority for some players or priority keeps changing

CHAPTER 4

Working with a medical writer

Professional medical writers are often involved in developing publications, especially those reporting industry-funded research. Some investigators and journal editors are uncomfortable about this practice, considering that it may encourage undue influence by the trial sponsor in presenting the results and introducing bias or may lead to problems of **ghost** and **guest authorship**. However, others recognise professional writers as facilitators who can raise the standard of publications and make the whole process simpler and quicker.

Having spent over 15 years earning my living as a medical writer, it will not be hard for readers to work out which view I believe is correct. However, in this chapter I will attempt to suppress my prejudices and consider the potential benefits and disadvantages of involving a professional writer.

■ Advantages of involving a medical writer

A good writer will bring the following skills and attributes to a project:

- excellent command of English
- expertise in preparing publications and presenting scientific data
- familiarity with journal requirements and preferences
- realistic ideas about chances of acceptance at different journals
- familiarity with guidelines such as **CONSORT, International Committee of Medical Journal Editors (ICMJE)** Uniform Requirements, **Good Publication Practice (GPP)** for pharmaceutical companies
- experience of dealing with journals, e.g. responding to reviewers' comments
- coordination and project management skills
- expertise in preparing **figures** or professional contacts for getting this done
- access to tools that make writing easier, e.g. software for creating references
- uninterrupted time to write (unlike most busy clinicians, a writer can offer dedicated writing time rather than having to fit writing around other commitments – this alone can often accelerate a project)
- ability to take an objective view of data – it is sometimes easier for an outsider

to assess results and, in particular, focus a publication by deciding what to leave out, than for the researcher who has lived with the work for some time.

Being an outsider (i.e. someone who has not taken part in the research), the writer may also be more aware of differences of opinion within the group than the members themselves (who have grown accustomed to each other's idiosyncrasies). The process of briefing a writer may also provide a focus for discussing all the elements of the publication (e.g. **journal choice, key messages**) which might otherwise not be discussed (since junior members of the group might accept suggestions from more senior members without challenging them). A full-time writer may also have more experience than the team members in preparing publications and therefore be able to advise on strategy and how to avoid common pitfalls.

■ Disadvantages of involving a medical writer

- *Money*: somebody has to pay the writer. This can cause problems if you have no budget for this or if the payment links the writer too strongly with the sponsor.
- *Lack of specialist knowledge*: most medical writers are generalists, they cannot be specialists in every field; however they are experts in presenting data and preparing publications. This means that you should not expect the writer to be familiar with the complete literature around a subject. Some writers do specialise and develop considerable knowledge in certain areas, or may be familiar with the literature from having recently prepared a related article, but you should not assume this.
- *Acknowledgement*: in most cases when a writer works from a study report, or prepares an outline and then a draft only after discussion with the investigators, the writer will not meet the ICMJE criteria for authorship, since s/he will not have been involved in study design, data collection, analysis or interpretation. However, the last category is open to a range of interpretation, and, if writers get involved early in a study (e.g. in writing the protocol) or work from data tables rather than a report, then they might qualify for authorship. This may raise questions about how the writer is acknowledged. If the **target journal** lists individuals' contributions to a study (rather than a traditional author list), omitting the writer from the list might raise queries from the editor, especially if this means that the person who prepared the first draft is not included in the list of **contributors/authors**. I personally feel it is quite acceptable for a medical writer to prepare a first draft of a paper and not to qualify as an author, since I prefer to apply the general rule about authors taking public responsibility for research, rather than the criteria of exactly who did what. However, some journal editors may consider that this is **ghost authorship**.

■ Other points to consider

The job description 'medical writer' should not be interpreted too narrowly – some of the skills that a professional writer brings to a writing group are those of project management and coordination. A good writer will be able to guide discussions at writing group meetings, ensure that all the issues (e.g. target journal, **order of authors**) have been addressed, and help the group achieve consensus. This coordinating role can be particularly helpful when authors are unable to meet because of distance or time constraints.

Paradoxically, authors and other writing group members will probably get the most from working with a professional writer if they remember the writer's limitations. Medical writers are usually good communicators with a broad biomedical background. They are not specialists and they are not telepathic. Time spent briefing the writer in the early stages is always a good investment. This process, in itself, may also be helpful, since it provides an opportunity for the group to discuss the important elements (such as key messages and target audience) together. Such discussion might not take place at all if the principal investigator prepares a draft and simply circulates it to all authors for comments.

For this reason (whether a writer is involved or not), it is usually a good idea to circulate an outline before preparing a draft. When working with a professional writer, the authors need to provide especially detailed input to the Introduction and Discussion sections. If the key messages have been agreed, and a detailed protocol and data tables are available, the writer should be able to produce a competent first draft of the Methods and Results without much assistance, but it is unrealistic to expect a writer alone to develop the other sections which require a detailed knowledge of the existing literature and an understanding of the clinical implications of the findings.

Once a draft has been circulated, it is usually the writer's task to collate comments. The simplest method is often to use the 'Track Changes' function on your word processor. This not only highlights the changes but indicates who has made them. However, if changes are extensive the resulting draft can get very messy and hard to read. Also, most software is not good at showing where sentences or paragraphs have simply been re-ordered, since there is no way of distinguishing a moved paragraph from one that has been rewritten. Specialized publication planning software may also be used to collate comments via a web-based system.

It may be possible for the writer to prepare a revised draft, incorporating all the comments, which is acceptable to all the authors. However, circulating drafts may reveal more fundamental differences in interpreting results, or varying views about how findings should best be presented. In this case, it is unreasonable to expect the writer to act as arbitrator. The best course is for the authors to settle their differences amongst themselves and then report the outcome to the writer. Similarly, it is unfair to expect writers to act as mediators in disagreements between sponsors and investigators.

CHAPTER 5

Dr Seymour and the disappearing paper: a cautionary tale

One stormy evening three shadowy figures emerged from a brooding tower overlooking a fetid swamp. Together they had hatched a plot to study Horrormycin, the latest product to emerge from the bubbling laboratories of the Darke Drug Corporation. These three schemers were Dr Procter, an ambitious medic, Mrs Countem, a buxom statistician, and Miss Plannem, a lowly study manager. Through mystical powers of telepathy and technology they had also consulted the sagely Professor Knowitall and the wealthy but indolent Dr Donothing. After days locked in the smoke-filled labyrinth they blinked in the weak November twilight, their weariness masked by the smug feeling that they had produced a masterly protocol for a study that would guarantee the success of Horrormycin.

After much grinding and refining in the forges of the legal and regulatory gnomes, the protocol was polished to perfection and the study began. (As this is a fairy story, it takes place in an allegorical land which did not have research ethics committees.)

Three months later, Professor Knowitall was struck by the palsy and retired to his castle. In March, Dr Procter met an awfully nice chap on the golf course who told him about a job at Potions Inc. offering twice his current salary, so he left the Darke Corporation. And, being spring time, Mr Countem felt the sap rise in his veins, and soon Mrs Countem was on maternity leave.

As autumn approached and the leaves began to fall, the study ended. Miss Plannem, who had managed to keep the study within budget, was rewarded by promotion to a different department, based in a distant land. The data were analysed, in Mrs Countem's absence, by the inscrutable Dr Chi. Medical queries were handled in a desultory manner by the younger but even more ambitious Dr Climber, who was now responsible for Horrormycin but whose main passion was Bustergut, rapidly emerging as a panacea that could make the Darke Corporation rich beyond even the wildest dreams of its directors. The job of preparing the study report from Dr Chi's inscrutable, and somewhat incomprehensible, statistics was given to humble Miss Tidy, a graduate who had only recently joined the corporation and knew little about Horrormycin and even less about statistics. She was terrified of Dr Climber and soon learnt that he did not like being bothered with trivial queries, even on the rare occasions when he was in his office, so she kept them to herself and grew increasingly pale and thin in her solitary labours, and resolved to escape back to the happier land of Academia as soon as she could.

Dr Climber realised that a publication would enhance his reputation, and had grown to despise the snivelling Miss Tidy, so he hired Ms Literate from the Ritemmup Agency for this task. However, Dr Climber was a busy man, and the Agency offices happened to be on his way to the golf course, so he simply flung the report at Ms Literate, along with a bag of gold, and demanded that she should produce a draft by the end of the week. He zoomed away on his corporate charger and soon was far too many leagues away to hear her plaintive wailing about identifying authors and journals.

As the conference season was approaching, Dr Donothing, who had failed to recruit a single patient to the study, sent smoke signals to Dr Climber, indicating that a trip to Costlyville would be most acceptable. Dr Climber was happy to agree (as he had also heard good reports about the Costlyville golf courses) but suggested his old friend Professor Regionale should be an author, as he had recruited one patient to the study, lived near Costlyville and might introduce him to the best golf club. Sadly, the smoke signals took a long time to reach Dr Climber and, by the time he replied, the deadline for submitting abstracts had passed, but this meant that the three men could enjoy the meeting (and the golf courses) without the tiresome distraction of making a presentation.

Meanwhile, in the cobweb-festooned corridors of Ritemmup, the paper progressed slowly and made many journeys back and forth to the caverns of marketing which lurked underneath Darke Towers. After the sixth round of comments, the owner of Ritemmup growled that the bag of gold would not cover any further embellishments and that it was time to get some authors for the paper. Dr Climber therefore sent the draft to Professor Regionale and also to Dr Seymour, a struggling young British doctor picked at random from the list of investigators because his name came after Professor Regionale's.

Honest Dr Seymour was surprised to receive the manuscript, since, despite recruiting several patients, he had never been told how the study had gone, so he asked for the original report. Dr Climber was glad to find somebody who took such an interest in the findings, but less delighted when Dr Seymour spotted a major problem with the analysis (caused by the inscrutable Dr Chi reading some tables from right to left, which had been overlooked by Miss Tidy). Fortunately, by this time, Mrs Countem had returned and, together with Dr Seymour, helped Ms Literate to prepare a totally revised version (but only after another bag of gold had been delivered to the agency).

The revised version was then sent to Dr Donothing, Professor Regionale and, at the suggestion of the marketing department, Dr Keen and Professor Igor, who lived in rich countries ravaged by disfiguring diseases that responded to Horrormycin. All except Dr Donothing added some comments and suggested changes to the paper, blissfully unaware of the original intentions of the study, and of the fact that the draft was now at least 1000 words over the limit for any journal. But Ms Literate applied her magic red quill pen, and produced another version. This was delivered, on a silver salver, to Dr Darke, the company's ageing and increasingly erratic founder, who invited the equally venerable and absent-minded Professor Importante to join the author list. Professor Importante could not remember if she had ever heard of this study, but she did not like to refuse her old friend. The paper descended once more into the vaults of the regulatory and legal gnomes and was finally submitted to the *Ivory Tower Journal of Impressive Results.*

The final list of authors was: Donothing, Regionale, Keen, Igor, Seymour, Climber and Importante. Somebody had found a yellowed parchment which stated that no more than one corporation employee could be included on any publication, so Mrs Countem was omitted in favour of the more persuasive and influential Dr Climber.

Meanwhile, unbeknown to Dr Climber, Dr Enthusiastikov, head of the Placebo Institute of Malpractica, which had recruited an unfeasibly large number of patients (many of whom were omitted from the main analysis since they failed to meet the inclusion criteria), had analysed the data from his institute. He submitted a paper (in the Malpractican dialect) to the *Journal of Salami Science* with himself as sole author and no mention of the Darke Corporation or the rest of the study because he had heard nothing from the Darke Corporation since the study ended, there was nothing in his contract to suggest he should not do this, and he was keen to enrich his CV with another publication.

By a strange stroke of fate, the *Ivory Tower Journal of Impressive Results* sent the paper to somebody who had already reviewed Dr Enthusiastikov's paper for the *JSS*, and she pointed out the similarities.

By this time, Dr Climber had lost all interest in Horrormycin and was devoting himself to Bustergut. He ignored Ms Literate's messages about the journal's concerns and concentrated on his golf handicap. Mrs Countem was disgruntled and unwilling to help, having been omitted from the author list and, as usual, Dr Donothing did nothing. A few months later, the Darke Corporation was swallowed up by Dragontooth Pharma, who stopped the development of Horrormycin, refused to give the Ritemmup Agency any more gold and sacked Mrs Countem as they disapproved of working mothers.

Dr Seymour was sorry that the study never got published, as he continued to see patients disfigured by infections that might have been cured by Horrormycin, but he was so busy administering other salves and potions that he soon forgot about it.

However, there is one magic formula guaranteed to stop papers from disappearing. It is called a 'Publication Strategy'. As with any form of magic, it can be used for both good and evil, and is a powerful force. Consult the rest of this book to discover how to achieve a good one!

Part Two

A to Z of
Publication Strategy

A

■ Abstracts

■ For conferences

Submission deadlines for abstracts to major conferences are non-negotiable. Organisers of smaller meetings occasionally extend their deadlines if they have not received as many abstracts as they hoped for, but you should never bank on this. If you have a really good reason why you cannot meet the deadline (e.g. your results will be available only a few days later) or you have good links or influence with the organising committee (e.g. you are working for one of the meeting's major sponsors) it might be worth contacting the organisers well before the deadline to see if there is any flexibility. But, in most cases, you will need to plan carefully to ensure you meet the deadline.

Despite their brevity, a lot can go wrong with abstracts, especially those that are submitted electronically on behalf of other people.

Tips to avoid delays and nervous breakdowns when submitting abstracts

Check the conference website well in advance for requirements such as:

- having abstracts sponsored by a member of the organising association
- limiting the number of abstracts each member can submit or sponsor
- limiting the number of abstracts on which an individual can be listed as first author.

In addition, check practical requirements such as:

- word limit
- whether tables are permitted
- preferred structure/headings.

Find out what author details are required, then obtain these well in advance. Details you might have forgotten could include:

- middle names/initials
- full postal address of institution
- telephone number (for presenting/first author)
- fax number (for presenting/first author)
- e-mail address (for all authors)
- membership number/name as it appears in the membership directory for sponsor

---

> - authors' dates of birth (especially if they are eligible for 'young presenter' awards)
> - any other obscure facts about the authors that you are unlikely to know (I recently heard of a conference website that required the authors' passport numbers).
>
> Also check what other decisions you will need to make. Make sure you discuss these with all authors and key players:
>
> - key words
> - topic/area of presentation (often selected from a list of sessions)
> - presentation preference (oral/poster).

As with any publication, allow sufficient time to get approval from all co-authors, your boss/institution and funding body, as appropriate.

Since an abstract is often the first publication to be developed from a research project, it is often the first document in which the authors are listed. A looming deadline is not conducive to rational and even-tempered discussion about author inclusion or order, so get this agreed well in advance (*see* **authorship** for guidance on this).

The principles of authorship used by journals generally apply to conference abstracts (although conference websites rarely bother to mention this). However, there is no absolute rule stating that the order of authors on an abstract must be identical to that on the final paper and it is acceptable to include local authors if they are presenting the findings at regional meetings.

While electronic submission makes some aspects easier, it also brings its own problems. Watch out for the following.

- The system used on the website to calculate the number of words will not necessarily produce the same figure as your software; be prepared to make last-minute adjustments if you are up to the word limit.
- Some websites will not accept unusual characters (e.g. Greek letters), symbols (e.g. ±), or foreign accents; consider using alternatives, e.g. mcg instead of µg, ae for German ä, etc.
- Even if websites appear to accept unusual characters, try to check their final appearance as they sometimes get garbled (e.g. Greek µ can turn into m with drastic consequences for drug doses).
- Increasing traffic as the deadline approaches may make websites slow to respond or even unworkable. Aim to submit your abstract as early as possible to avoid the rush.

If you know you will have to submit an abstract close to the deadline and perhaps without time to contact the authors about last-minute queries it is a good idea to do a 'dummy submission'. Many websites only allow you to see all the pages (and therefore discover what information is required) once you have started a submission, so it makes sense to have a trial run going through all the pages just up to the actual submission. This will show you exactly what you need for the submission and should avoid last-minute hitches.

Try to agree the contents in good time with all the authors. Discussing the **key messages** of the research will be time well spent, since you can often only squeeze one or two major outcomes into an abstract.

Unlike papers, rules about multiple publication do not apply. You may therefore split your findings over several abstracts (e.g. one on safety, one on efficacy, one on a sub-group analysis). You may also submit similar abstracts to several meetings (unless a conference accepts only new data). In general, the largest (US and international) meetings will not accept findings that have been presented elsewhere. It therefore pays to plan your meetings carefully, if necessary reserving the first presentation for a large meeting, and using smaller, national or regional meetings for secondary presentations. Including trial registration numbers on abstracts (as recommended by CONSORT for Abstracts) should make it clear when several presentations relate to the same study and help to link abstracts to full papers.

Abstracts submitted to meetings do not affect later submissions of full reports to journals. However, see the section on **prior publication** for more details.

■ Of a paper

The abstract is a crucial part of the paper and, in many cases, the only part that gets read. This means it must be accurate, and it ought to be sufficiently interesting to entice your audience to read the rest of the paper. Some journal editors perform their initial screening by reading only the abstract. An announcement in the *BMJ* contained the advice: 'Please get the abstract right, because we may use it alone to assess your paper'.

The easiest time to write the abstract is after you have written the rest of the paper. Check the journal's instructions for word limits and structure. If the journal does not stipulate a structure, consider using headings as they improve readability.

Abstract headings are usually similar to those in the main body of the text, i.e. Introduction (or Background, or Objectives), Methods, Results, Conclusion (or Discussion).

Most journals limit the size of abstracts and indexing services may truncate abstracts. For example, **Medline** used to cut abstracts off after 250 words even if a longer version appeared in the journal. However, the Medline limit is now 10 000 characters (or about 1000 words) so, in practice, this isn't usually a problem. Try to follow CONSORT for abstracts which provides a useful checklist on the content.

Although it may be tempting to leave writing the abstract until a late draft of the paper, do not leave it too late. All authors should have sufficient time to comment on this important section of the paper. However, remember to update the abstract whenever other parts of the paper are changed. The abstract should never contain findings that do not appear in the main text. Round up numbers consistently so that figures in the main text and abstract are identical. If a figure can sensibly be rounded up in the abstract, consider rounding it up elsewhere. Strings of decimal places reduce readability and often do not add anything meaningful.

Groves T and Abbasi K (2004) Screening research papers by reading abstracts. *BMJ. 329*: 470–1.

Hopewell S, Clarke M, Moher D, Wager E *et al* (2008) CONSORT for reporting randomised trials in journal and conference abstracts. *Lancet* **371**: 281–3.

■ Acceptance rates

■ Journals

These range from 5–85% and should therefore be a major factor when selecting a target journal. Well-known general journals such as *The Lancet* and *The New England Journal of Medicine (NEJM)* reject over 90% of the papers they receive, while new, electronic journals or those operating a 'bias to publish' reject only around 15%. Some journals publish their acceptance statistics each year and others give some idea of this on their websites or in their 'Instructions to authors'. If you cannot find the precise figure, assume:

- prestigious general journals 5–20%
- prestigious specialist journals 10–30%
- other specialist journals 30–50%
- new titles, obscure journals 40–70%
- **pay journals** 70–90%.

Submitting to a journal with a frighteningly low acceptance rate may not be a bad strategy, but you should always have a **back-up plan** in case you are rejected, and you should think about what effects rejection might have on your timetable (*see* **acceptance times** and **rejection times**).

■ Meetings

These are generally much higher than for journals; 50–70% is not uncommon. However, unlike journals, many conferences do not publicise their acceptance rates so they can be hard to ascertain. Since you may submit similar abstracts to several meetings, their acceptance rates need not concern you as much as journals when planning a publication strategy.

■ Acceptance times

The time from submission to acceptance varies enormously between journals so this will be an important criterion for selection if speed is important. Many journals give some idea of decision times in their 'Instructions to authors', but bear in mind that these may be averages or even optimistic targets (beware of phrases such as 'we aim to give a decision in four weeks . . .'). Some helpful journals publish their actual performance statistics each year.[1] Others give information about acceptance times by publishing submission and acceptance dates on each article. In other cases, ask a colleague who has submitted something to the journal in the last few years.

Bear in mind that time to acceptance is often longer than time to rejection, especially in journals that reject a large proportion of papers after in-house review. Time to acceptance also includes the time taken by authors to respond to reviewers' comments (which journal editors delight in reminding us can be lengthy) and time for additional rounds of review.

1 For example, Fontanarosa PB and DeAngelis CD (2009) Thank you, JAMA peer reviewers and authors. *JAMA*. **301**: 870.

See also **rejection times** and Chapter 3 'How long will it take?' (pp. 13–16).

■ Access to data

Good Publication Practice recommends that 'sponsors have a responsibility to share the data and the analyses with the investigators who participated in the study'. This responsibility should be set out in the **publication agreement**.
See also **Ownership of data.**

■ Acknowledgements
■ People

Some journals, for example *JAMA* and *Annals of Internal Medicine*, require the corresponding author to state that written confirmation has been received from everybody mentioned in the acknowledgements. It is therefore a good idea to include the acknowledgements in an early draft so that you are not delayed by gathering the confirmations. Even if journals do not require written confirmation, it is only polite to inform anybody you plan to acknowledge and you should respect their request if they prefer not to be named. Use the acknowledgements section to thank people who have helped the project, but do not merit authorship, such as investigators outside the writing group, study nurses, data monitors and medical writers or author's editors.

Check journal instructions to see what roles can be acknowledged. Although acknowledgements are generally used to record the contributions of medical writers who do not fulfil the **International Committee of Medical Journal Editors' (ICMJE)** criteria for authorship, a few journals, notably *Neurology*, insist that 'professional writers employed by pharmaceutical companies . . . who have drafted or revised the intellectual content of the paper must be included as authors'.

■ Funding

The source of funding or support for research (including writing assistance) should always be described. Many journals include funding details in the acknowledgements section, but some put this information in a footnote on the title page, or in the methods. It is good practice to include some kind of **trial identification**, such as a trial registration number. Identifying the trial helps people preparing systematic reviews and may discourage **redundant publication**. Members of the **ICMJE** have required trial registration as a condition for publication in their journals since July 2005 and many other journals have followed their lead.

DeAngelis C, Drazen JM, Frizelle FA *et al* (2004) Clinical trial registration: a statement from the International Committee of Medical Journal Editors. *Lancet* **364**: 911–2

Wager E (2004) The need for trial identifiers. *Curr Med Res Opin*. **20**: 203–6.

■ Advertising departments

If you want detailed information about who reads a journal and where these readers work, the best source is the advertising department (if the journal has one). This department uses the information to persuade customers to place advertisements in the journal. If the journal does not carry display advertisements, you could try contacting the editorial office or subscriptions department, but they may not have the information in such detail or it may be difficult to find the correct person to speak to.

■ Affiliations; *see author affiliations*

■ American Medical Writers Association (AMWA)

This organisation produces a code of conduct for medical writers and has issued a position statement on their involvement with publications.[1] Its European sister organisation, the European Medical Writers Association (EMWA), has also produced a statement (*see* Appendix 3, pp. 139–45).[2]

1 http://www.amwa.org/default.asp?Mode=DirectoryDisplay&id=223

2 Jacobs A and Wager E (2005) EMWA guidelines on the role of medical writers in developing peer-reviewed publications. *Curr Med Res Opin*. **21**(2): 317–21.

■ Anonymous reviewers

Most journals do not disclose the identity of reviewers to authors. Anonymity is supposed to enable reviewers to speak their mind without fearing the consequences. Its supporters claim that anonymity overcomes the problem of junior scientists being unwilling to criticise the work of more senior researchers for fear of damaging their careers. However, a few journals have challenged this idea and now practise 'open reviewing', arguing that it is fairer if authors know the identity of their reviewers. The *BMJ* studied the effects of open review before adopting it. The studies found that open review was feasible (i.e. only a tiny proportion of reviewers refused to sign), but had little discernible effect on review quality or tone. This should reassure those who feared that reviewers would be reluctant to criticise work if they knew their name would be revealed to authors. However, it does not support the opposing view that open review would produce more detailed, or more courteous, reviews.

Even if the journal does not reveal reviewers' names, many authors think they can guess their reviewers' identity, but they are often wrong.[1] It is therefore unwise to bear a lifelong grudge against somebody you suspect of reviewing your work harshly; it was probably somebody else.

Journals that reveal reviewers' names to authors definitely do not like authors to contact the reviewers directly, even if that seems the simplest way to resolve a disagreement. You should always address reviewers' comments via the editor.

Some journals ask authors to suggest potential reviewers, or allow them to indicate if there is anybody they do not want as a reviewer (*see* **reviewer choice**). However, unless the journal practises open review you may never know if your suggestions were adopted.

Some journals take anonymity one stage further by trying to mask the authors' identity – *see* **blinded (masked) review** for more details.

1 Wesseley S *et al* (1996) Do authors know who refereed their paper? A questionnaire survey. *BMJ*. **313**: 1185.

■ Appeals

A rejection is always disappointing, and fighting it may be a natural reaction, but it is usually better to swallow your pride and switch to your **back-up plan**. However, there are a few circumstances when it may be worth appealing. One is when you receive at least one favourable review, but the journal editor seems to be swayed by a single negative review. If you can give objective reasons why the negative reviewer is wrong, or demonstrates bias, it may be worth sending a carefully worded letter to the editor. Unless you know the editor well, you should not telephone, as most editors will consider only written appeals. Before you appeal, look carefully at the editor's letter for clues about the reason for rejection. If the editor indicates that your submission is not suited to the journal, there is little point in appealing, even if some of the reviewers' comments are favourable.

The *BMJ*'s 'Instructions to Contributors' advises: 'Appeals clarifying and revising specific parts of the manuscript, for instance the analysis of original data, tend to succeed much more often than appeals against essentially editorial decisions. If the editors and/or the full editorial committee have decided that your paper is not sufficiently interesting or important for *BMJ* readers, there may be no point in trying to appeal'. The *BMJ* also points out that 'we can consider only one appeal per manuscript. Our experience is that prolonged negotiations over rejected papers are usually unsatisfactory for both authors and editors.'[1]

If you feel that a journal has mistreated you in some way, other than by simply not recognising the brilliance of your work, you should write to the editor or, if the journal has one, the **ombudsman/ombudsperson**. Alerting the editor to your grievance may not undo the damage but it might help other authors by preventing future problems, and getting the matter off your chest may be therapeutic. Many journals track reviewer performance so a letter from an author might encourage the editor to avoid that reviewer in future.

The **Committee on Publication Ethics (COPE)** considers cases brought by journal editors which may involve misconduct by authors or reviewers. However, COPE does not consider cases from aggrieved authors about editorial decisions. If you feel you have not got a satisfactory response from the editor, you could approach the journal's governing body, especially if this is an academic society, or the publisher. The **World Association of Medical Editors (WAME)** has an ethics committee that considers cases from members, not all of whom are journal editors, so this might offer a possible avenue for complaint.

Whatever you do, make sure you do not spend so much energy on your grievances and appeals that you have none left to implement your **back-up plan**.

1 http://bmj.bmjjournals.com/advice/article_submission.shtml

■ Artwork; *see* figure legends; figures; graphs

■ Author affiliations

List the affiliations of authors at the time they did the study. This helps readers understand where the work was done and credits the institutions. If authors have changed jobs since the research was done you may also include their current affiliation. Ask all authors to check their details on the very first draft they see; do not wait until just before submission. Check with your institution for the correct way of naming it. If in doubt, check your payslip or headed notepaper to find the formal name of your employer. For example, for UK National Health Service (NHS) hospitals this is usually the name of the trust, rather than the more familiar name of a single hospital or clinic.

■ Authorship

The authorship of publications can cause many headaches. The two important rules are to:

• be familiar with recognised authorship criteria, for example those from the **International Committee of Medical Journal Editors (ICMJE)**
• discuss authorship early in the research process.

The ICMJE states that authors should be able to take public responsibility for the research and the publication. This normally involves contributing to study design or interpretation, as well as playing an active part in developing the publication and approving the final version.

Some journals have abandoned the traditional author **by-line** for the **contributorship** system where individuals' contributions to the research are listed. Check which system your **target journal** uses. Also consult the sections on the **writing group**, **number of authors** and **order of authors**. To understand problems to avoid, *see* **ghost author(s)** and **guest authors/gift authorship** and read the tale of 'Dr Seymour and the disappearing paper' (pp. 21–24).

For further reading try:

Albert T and Wager E (2003) How to handle authorship disputes: a guide for new researchers. *COPE Report 2003*. Committee on Publication Ethics, London. www.publicationethics.org.uk

B

■ Back-up plan

Selecting a **target journal** is not always easy because the **key players** may have different aims and expectations. For example, speed of publication may be the most important criterion for one person, while journal **impact factor** may be more important to another.

Since many journals have high rejection rates, and since it can take time to get agreement about the target journal, it is always a good idea to have a back-up plan and to select a second journal in case your paper is rejected by the first. If you do not select the second journal at the same time as the first, you may miss an opportunity for discussion and waste a lot of time. A rejection is always unwelcome and, even if it is not entirely unexpected, it often leads to loss of motivation and momentum and thus further delay.

Choosing a second target journal may also help to meet varied expectations. For example, if some authors are keen to aim for a prestigious journal, while others are more concerned about rapid publication, you might agree to submit first to a prestigious journal that uses **in-house review** and therefore has short rejection times, but agree to submit to a less prestigious journal with a greater chance of acceptance, and/or reasonably rapid publication, if your paper is rejected by the first.

■ Bias

Scientists and clinicians are expected to have opinions about what their findings mean but they are also expected to present results fairly and responsibly. As with many ethical questions it is hard to provide a working definition of bias but the following examples of biased reporting give ideas about what to avoid.

Examples of reporting bias

- Presenting secondary or *post hoc* analyses as if they were the primary endpoints of a study if the primary endpoints did not turn out as you had hoped.
- 'Cherry picking' the most favourable endpoints or test results and omitting others that do not fit your hypothesis (e.g. reporting six-month efficacy data but omitting 12-month results because they do not reach statistical significance, or reporting results of one rating scale but not another).
- Omitting adverse events or clumping them into meaningless categories (e.g. not detailing the number of deaths but including these among all serious adverse events).
- Failing to describe a study population adequately if some special features of this population might affect the results (e.g. reporting treatment preference without mentioning that patients had previously failed on another therapy).

■ 'Big Five'

- *Annals of Internal Medicine*
- *BMJ (British Medical Journal)*
- *JAMA (Journal of the American Medical Association)*
- *The Lancet*
- *New England Journal of Medicine (NEJM)*

are sometimes known, informally, as the 'Big Five'. All but *Annals* are weekly, and they all have large subscription bases. They are all represented on the **International Committee of Medical Journal Editors** (ICMJE, or Vancouver Group) and have been influential in developing peer-review research and policy. Many studies of peer-review practices have focused on the big five, which is a pity, since, although they are undoubtedly influential, they are also atypical. Unlike smaller journals run by academic societies, the big five have full-time editors and large numbers of editorial staff. This means they reject up to 50% of submissions after internal review. They also tend to invest quite heavily in **technical editing**, so, if your paper is accepted, you can expect it to be knocked pretty firmly into **house style**. The big five is a purely subjective grouping and some of the larger specialty journals (such as *Circulation* and *Neurology*) operate in similar ways. However, such big journals do operate differently from those with part-time, academic editors, and you should bear this in mind when dealing with them.

■ BioMed Central

A series of electronic **Open Access journals**. They have some innovative features including open peer review, publishing reviewers' comments alongside papers, and requiring authors to suggest potential reviewers. They also require that all randomised trials be entered into a trial register or given a unique **ISRCTN** (**International Standard Randomised Controlled Trial Number**) identifier. Not to be confused with **PubMed Central**.

See www.biomedcentral.com

■ Blinded (masked) review

Several studies have attempted to test whether it matters if reviewers know the identity of the authors. Overall, the results are inconclusive, with some studies showing an effect and others not. The idea behind blinded review is that reviewers may be prejudiced by the authors' prestige, or lack of it. One study examined this by sending two versions of the same paper to several reviewers. In one version, the authors were from prestigious institutions, while in the second version the authors came from a fictitious (and unimpressive-sounding) centre. Reviewers apparently demonstrated institutional bias by criticising the paper from the prestigious institution less harshly. However, other studies have shown the opposite effect, with well-known authors receiving tougher reviews than junior scientists. Studies have also shown that it is difficult to mask authors' identities effectively because authors tend to cite their own work and reviewers often recognise researchers in their own field.

As an author, the only choice you have about whether your identity will be revealed to the reviewer, or whether the journal will reveal the reviewers' identity to you, is your choice of target journal (*see* **anonymous reviewers** for more details). If you feel strongly about this you may be able to discover the journal's methods in the 'Instructions to authors' guidance notes; but don't bank on it.

If you choose a journal that uses blinded review, try to facilitate this by putting all the author details on a separate title page and making sure author names do not appear in the filename or as a header or footer. For obvious reasons ophthalmology journals tend to use the term 'masked review' in preference to 'blinded'.

■ Books

Primary publications of research should appear in peer-reviewed journals rather than books because journal articles generally take less time to be published and are searchable via indexing and abstracting systems. However, book chapters often provide useful subject reviews and may provide greater freedom in terms of length, scope and format than journals. A book is an excellent format if your aim is primarily to educate or entertain your readers. I hope that this one succeeds in doing a little of both.

■ By-line (or masthead)

Policies on authorship in journals are far less uniform than the **International Committee of Medical Journal Editors' (ICMJE)** 'Uniform Requirements for Manuscripts Submitted to Biomedical Journals' might suggest. *See* **authorship** and **contributorship (vs. authorship)** for more detailed discussions of these concepts. The by-line is a convenient place to set out various options and mention related issues.

Before the late 1990s, journals simply listed authors and their affiliations. This listing was equivalent to the by-line (or masthead) in a newspaper, which tells readers who an article is by. However, some journals now publish details of who did what. This list of contributors usually appears separately from the list of authors and so, in theory, it is possible for the contributor list to be different from the by-line. Although a few journals will permit it, having different individuals listed as authors and contributors is likely to raise questions about how **authorship** was allocated.

Further variation in practice occurs in how journals regard group names. Some will permit the formula 'Crank & Bloggs on behalf of the Whizzo Study Group' without the entire study group being listed, and without all the individual members of the study group fulfilling the journal's authorship criteria. However, other journals make a stricter interpretation of the by-line and insist that all members of a group are listed (for example in a footnote) and that all members meet authorship criteria.

For more information *see* **names**.

C

■ Checklists

Some journals include a checklist for submission within their instructions to contributors. What you need to submit depends on the journal. If your target journal provides a checklist, then follow it. If it does not, consider the following:

- **covering letter** – this should include a statement that the work is original and is not being considered for publication elsewhere
- authors' signatures/author declaration – stating that they have contributed to the publication and approved its submission
- authors' declarations of competing interests/financial support
- **copyright** transfer document – some journals require authors to relinquish copyright to the publisher – usually the corresponding author has to sign this
- authorisation from people mentioned in the **acknowledgements** or quoted as **personal communications**
- evidence that references cited as being 'in press' have been accepted for publication

- **permissions** to reproduce figures or tables from other publications
- consent from patients to publish personal details, e.g. in case studies.

■ ClinicalTrials.gov

This is a trial register sponsored by the United States National Library of Medicine. For more details look at www.clinicaltrials.gov. In September 2004, the **International Committee of Medical Journal Editors** announced that **trial registration** would be a condition for publication in their journals after July 2005.[1] At that time, only ClinicalTrials.gov met the editors' criteria but, since then, ICMJE has recognized other registers.

A US law, passed in 2007, made registration in ClinicalTrials.gov compulsory for most clinical trials. *See* **FDAAA** for more details. This Act also required study results to be posted on ClinicalTrials.gov so it has become a results repository as well as a trial register. Not to be confused with www.clinicaltrialresults.org (a sort of Wiki for results, set up by researchers) or www.clinicalstudyresults.org (a results website run by **Pharmaceutical Research and Manufacturers of America (PhRMA)**.

1 DeAngelis C, Drazen JM, Frizelle FA *et al.* (2004) Clinical trial registration: a statement from the International Committee of Medical Journal Editors. *The Lancet.* **364**: 911–2.

■ Co-authors

If you are having trouble deciding who your co-authors should be, consult the sections on **authorship, order of authors**, and **number of authors**.

Remember to involve all authors as fully as possible when developing a publication plan and to consult them over all decisions, however minor. People can have strong feelings about the most unexpected aspects of publication strategy (*see* **expectations**). It is therefore remarkably easy for co-authors to fall out with or irritate each other.

If you develop a tough hide yourself, but assume that everybody else is likely to be injured by the slightest snub, you should survive, and might even live to work together on future projects. *See* **nitpickers** for hints on dealing with this particular species of co-author.

Remember that treating co-authors respectfully does not mean that you should be vague about what you want them to do. Clarity of communication is important, and it is always good to be explicit about deadlines and other requirements.

On a practical point, try to gather all the information you will need about your co-authors as early as possible. This may include full **names, author affiliations**, qualifications, contact details, membership of relevant organisations (if this is required to submit an abstract) and statements on **competing interests**.

■ Collaborators; *see group authorship*

■ Committee on Publication Ethics (COPE)

COPE was established by journal editors to provide help with ethical issues. The Committee discusses cases anonymously and then offers advice. COPE considers troublesome cases from editors but does not accept complaints from aggrieved authors. Cases are summarised in an annual report available at: www.publicationethics.org. COPE also publishes a code of conduct for editors and a series of flowcharts on how to handle suspected misconduct.

■ Competing interest; *see* conflicting interest

■ Conditional acceptance

This is the most common positive response you will receive from a journal. It does not mean that your submission has been accepted, but offers definite hope of acceptance if you can address the reviewers' concerns.

Some journals ask reviewers to indicate whether a submission should be accepted with minor modification or only after substantial revision. Most journals only give a conditional acceptance to the first category. If a major rewrite is required, you will probably be invited to resubmit (which is a bit worse than a conditional acceptance but still better than a rejection).

However, even though the requested changes may be relatively minor, the conversion rate between conditional and full acceptance does vary between journals, so you must be realistic. Discovering the odds of making the leap from conditional to full acceptance requires a good understanding of your target journal's peer-review process.

Journals fall into five categories.

1 *Journals with a 'bias to publish', or pay journals*: expect authors to make a reasonable attempt to answer reviewers' questions, but then accept virtually all submissions from those that do.
2 *Academic journals in which the editor makes the final decision based on the referees' reports*: expect authors to address referees' concerns or give reasons why they have not made any suggested changes, but probably accept most submissions that get favourable referees' reports without consulting the referees again.
3 *Academic journals in which the editor returns the revised submission to the reviewers*: in these journals your submission could be rejected if you cannot address all the reviewers' concerns.
4 *Journals in which the editor sends the revised version to a new reviewer*: this can be extremely frustrating, since the new reviewer may suggest quite different changes from the original ones. This sometimes feels like entering another review round and it is difficult to predict the likelihood of full acceptance.
5 *Journals where the final decision is made by the editorial board or a committee*: a con-

ditional acceptance from this type of journal has the lowest chance of turning into a full acceptance. For example, *The Lancet* accepts only about one-third of the papers that reach this stage, regardless of how thoroughly the authors have responded to the reviewers' comments. In effect, this committee stage represents a third hurdle for submissions. Not only does the submission have to fall within the scope of the journal (which is determined by in-house review), it also has to pass the scientific scrutiny of the reviewers (hurdle number two) and finally, to get published, it has to be one of the most interesting submissions reviewed by the committee.

So, your chance of full acceptance after receiving a conditional acceptance ranges from around 30% to over 90%, depending on the journal. The trick is to understand your target journal and therefore understand where you stand.

Of course, there are also other factors that may affect whether a conditional acceptance turns into a full one. If you refuse to follow the reviewers' and editor's recommendations your chances will be reduced. And, in some cases, reviewers impose conditions that are impossible for you to meet, for example, demanding data that you did not collect, or a further analysis that you are not prepared to do.

Remember that a conditional acceptance is not the same as a full acceptance, so you cannot cite your paper as being 'in press' until you get the final acceptance letter. Remember to build in time for responding to reviewers' comments, and possibly for a further round of review, if you are trying to work out how long the overall process to publication will take.

■ Conflict of interest / competing interest

The **International Committee of Medical Journal Editors' (ICMJE)** 'Uniform Requirements for Manuscripts Submitted to Biomedical Journals' defines conflict of interest as 'financial or personal relationships that inappropriately influence the actions of authors, editors or reviewers'. It also notes that the potential for conflict of interest can exist whether or not somebody believes that the relationship affects his or her scientific judgement. For this reason, the term 'potential conflicts of interest' is sometimes used. The World Association of Medical Editors (**WAME**) emphasizes the importance of perceptions about competing interests in its definition: 'Conflict of interest (COI) exists when there is a divergence between an individual's private interests (competing interests) and his or her responsibilities to scientific and publishing activities such that a reasonable observer might wonder if the individual's behavior or judgment was motivated by considerations of his or her competing interests'. Many journals now require authors (and reviewers) to declare their interests. Most concentrate on financial interests such as employment, consultancies, research funding and stock ownership. But the Uniform Requirements note that conflicts can occur for other reasons 'such as personal relationships, academic competition, and intellectual passion'. Some journals (and institutions such as the US Food and Drug Administration) have attempted to set thresholds for financial relationships, considering that owning half a dozen shares in a big company is different from owning half the company. But in most cases, it is up to the author to decide what to declare. A good rule is to think of the most cynical person imaginable, who will impute a bad motive wherever possible, and to ask yourself what he or she might consider could have influenced the conduct or reporting of your research.

Journal editors have focused increasingly on competing interests after some highly publicised cases where authors tried to conceal their connections with research sponsors, such as tobacco companies. This led some journals (e.g. the *NEJM*) to attempt to prevent people with any competing interests from writing editorials and reviews. However, many journals found this unworkable, since the best-qualified and most experienced people usually have some links with research sponsors, so most journals now define a significant or disqualifying interest, or simply have policies to encourage transparency. But check before you plan to write an editorial.

Over the years, journals have evolved their own standards and recommendations on disclosure thresholds. This led to a rather messy situation in which an author might be expected to disclose financial relationships over the life of a project for one journal, going back three years for another journal and five years in another – leading to apparent inconsistencies (and even cases in which authors who had simply followed a journal's rules were accused of covering up certain interests). In an attempt to impose uniformity, the ICMJE issued a uniform disclosure form in October 2009 (available at www.icmje.org/coi_disclosure.pdf). This will be used at ICMJE member journals and will be reviewed (and may be revised) in April 2010.[1]

Gather information about all authors' competing interests as soon as possible (don't wait until the pre-submission draft). Some journals provide a tick list, others leave authors to devise their own wording for the declaration. Including a competing interest statement in an early draft gives authors a chance to read what co-authors have written and may jog memories about things that ought to be declared, or suggest helpful wording or ways to present this information accurately but concisely.

There is no excuse for attempting to conceal a conflict of interest, but research suggests that declarations can influence readers' perceptions of a publication. Editors at the *BMJ* sent two versions of a paper to 300 subscribers. The only difference between the versions was that one stated the authors were employed by a fictitious drug company, while the other stated that the authors had no competing interests. The 170 readers who responded were not only more sceptical about the version with the competing interest, rating it as less believable and less valid than the one with untainted authors, but they also rated it as less interesting and less relevant.[2]

Decisions about authorship of publications reporting research should never be influenced by considerations about competing interests. If a company employee merits authorship, he or she should be listed. However, if you are planning a letter to the editor or an editorial you might consider whether involving an author with a strong competing interest could lessen its impact.

1 Drazen JM, Van Der Weyden MB, Sahni P *et al.* (2009) Uniform format for disclosure of competing interests in ICMJE journals. *NEJM* 10.1056/NEJMe0909052 www.nejm.org

2 Chaudhry S, Schroter S, Smith R *et al.* (2002) Does declaration of competing interests affect reader perceptions? A randomised trial. *BMJ.* **325**: 1391–2.

Gottlieb S (2002) *New England Journal* loosens its rules on conflict of interest. *BMJ.* **324**: 1474.

James A and Horton R (2003) *The Lancet*'s policy on conflicts of interest. *The Lancet*. **361**: 8–9.

Smith R (1998) Beyond conflict of interest. Transparency is the key. *BMJ*. **317**: 291–2.

■ Congress / conference choice

A quick scan of websites listing medical congresses shows a dizzying number, so how do you choose the right one(s) for presenting your work? Some of the factors you need to consider are essentially the same as for **target journals**, namely **target audience**, reputation and **acceptance rates**. In addition you need to consider the following.

- *Timing*:
    - can you produce your abstract to meet the submission deadline?
    - does the timing of the meeting suit your strategy? (e.g. to coincide with a product launch, or to ensure no interference with the main publication).
- *Location*: can you afford to attend (and, let's face it, is it somewhere you would like to go)? Will your institution/company let you attend? These days most companies not only have budgetary restrictions but may also have security considerations; even if these do not affect you directly they may affect other delegates, e.g. attendance at conferences in the Middle East, including Turkey, has dropped since 2001.
- *Cost*: as well as getting to the meeting, you need to budget for the conference fees, accommodation and the cost of producing a poster or slides.
- *Special requirements*: some meetings require abstracts to be sponsored by members of the organising society, or may restrict the number of abstracts each member can submit.
- *Congress accepting data that have been presented previously*: some major international and US meetings will accept only new data, but smaller meetings do not impose such restrictions. You might therefore choose to hold back your abstract from a major meeting to ensure that presentation at a smaller one will not jeopardise this. Most meetings do not accept data that have already been published in full.

It is acceptable to submit essentially the same abstract to several meetings, especially if participants come from different specialties or regions. However, you should avoid submitting multiple abstracts to meetings that are likely to have widely overlapping audiences, since participants may not share your enthusiasm for your research and probably will not appreciate seeing your results several times.

For information about what conferences are taking place do an internet search or refer to one of the many websites that offer this information such as: www.medical-conferences.com or the Congress Resource Center on www.docguide.com

For information about specific conferences, check their websites and ask people who have attended previous meetings. Colleagues may be your only source of information about the reputation of meetings, since, unlike journals, there are no **impact factors**. You could also search professional or topic-focused web-based discussion sites for opinions about what meetings are really like. Colleagues may also be the best source of information about acceptance rates, since congresses rarely publish these. However, since you can submit abstracts to several meetings at once, the acceptance rates are less crucial than for journals. Information about conferences is also commercially available from communication agencies or specialist providers such as **DataVision** and **PeerView**.

■ CONSORT

The CONSORT statement is a useful resource for anybody reporting results of randomised controlled trials. The recommendations were developed because published reports did not contain enough information for people preparing systematic reviews. The statement aims to be evidence-based and it has been adopted by several hundred journals. Even if you are submitting a paper to a journal that has not formally adopted the CONSORT statement it is a good idea to follow it. The accompanying checklist is helpful, especially if you have not written this sort of paper before. The statement contains a lot of detail on reporting statistical methods and has a strong emphasis on robust randomisation and methods of minimising bias. It recommends that reports should include a figure (often called a CONSORT diagram) showing what happened to patients during a trial. Although they tend to be published only for more complex studies, preparing such a diagram can be a useful exercise and help to resolve queries about vanishing patients. Submitting a CONSORT diagram with your paper (even though you don't expect it will be published) may also show that you are aware of the guidelines and followed them when you wrote your report.

The statement is available at www.consort-statement.org or www.equator-network.org (which is a useful site containing links to many reporting guidelines).

■ CONSORT for Abstracts

The most recent addition to the CONSORT family is a checklist of items to include when reporting randomised trials in abstracts for conferences or journal articles. It recommends including a trial registration number and details about study funding. Some, but by no means all, of the journals that have adopted the main CONSORT statement have also adopted these guidelines, so check the instructions. Realising that journals like to do their own thing, CONSORT for Abstracts does not stipulate the format or headings that the abstract should contain, so you also need to check individual journal and conference requirements for these. Including all the items in the checklist should make your abstract more useful to readers (including reviewers and editors) so it makes sense to follow the guidance even if the journal or congress doesn't explicitly require it (but I'm biased, as I helped develop the guideline!).

Hopewell S, Clarke M, Moher D, Wager E *et al.* (2008) CONSORT for reporting randomised trials in journal and conference abstracts. *Lancet* **371**: 281–3.

■ Contact details

Journals require full contact details for the **corresponding author**. This usually means full postal address, telephone and fax numbers, and e-mail address. Remember to inform the journal if any details change after submission, otherwise your notification of acceptance or proofs may go astray. If you are not the corresponding author, try to obtain these details on an early draft. It is bothersome to have to delay submission because you forgot to get the corresponding author's fax number (and s/he is guaranteed to be away when you need this urgently).

■ Contracts

Research is rarely a solo exercise and large projects virtually always involve some sort of relationship between a sponsor/funder and the investigator(s). The nature of this relationship should be set out in an **investigators' agreement** or contract.

The contract is an excellent place to record decisions about the planned publication strategy, but, sadly, many sponsors ignore this opportunity or include only minimal details. Many problems with publications arise because sponsor and investigator have not discussed the strategy or have different **expectations** about it. Such problems get harder to resolve if they are left until the end of a project. It therefore makes sense to discuss publication plans at the earliest stage and to get agreement before the contract is signed.

Although it will not be possible to determine who will qualify as an author before the research has started, it should be possible to set out principles about how a **writing group** will be constituted. It is never too early to start discussing this.

Contracts should include something about data ownership and data access. If you feel a proposed contract is unduly restrictive, get advice from your boss and/or institution. **Good Publication Practice (GPP)** for pharmaceutical companies states that companies should never attempt to **veto** publications, although they may, legitimately, ask to see a draft before submission, be given time to comment on it, and, in some circumstances, request a delay in publication to, for example, protect intellectual property rights. Some journals now ask authors to state whether they had free access to the data and how much control the sponsor had over the decision to publish.

Unfortunately there have been cases in which investigators signed restrictive contracts permitting sponsors to suppress a publication. In these cases, the investigators' institutions have been reluctant to defend their employees' right to publish, since they feared legal action. When such cases have come to light they have generated bad publicity for the companies involved. Two, well-publicised cases are those of Nancy Olivieri[1] and Betty Dong.[2]

1 *Olivieri case*: Spurgeon D (2001) Report clears researcher who broke drug company agreement. *BMJ*. **323**: 1085.

2 *Dong case*: Rennie D (1998) Thyroid storm. *JAMA*. **277**: 1238–43.

Recognising the problems that can occur if there is no contract, the 2009 update of GPP recommends written **publication agreements** (*see* Appendix 3, pp. 150–66).

■ Contributorship (vs. authorship)

Some journals (in particular, the **'Big Five'**) recognise that authorship of research papers is a complex, even messy, business and have therefore shifted from a system of authorship to one of contributorship. This is also reflected in the latest version of the **International Committee of Medical Journal Editors' (ICJME)** 'Uniform Requirements for Manuscripts Submitted to Biomedical Journals'. Instead of simply listing authors in the **by-line**, these journals provide an indication of each individual's contribution to the research and the publication. In recognition of the fact that each contributor may have had an input to only part of the project, these journals sometimes also require one contributor to act as **guarantor** for the project's overall integrity.

Authors/contributors therefore need to check the journal's requirements to see what information is required. If you plan to submit to a journal that lists contributors and their contributions, gather this information as soon as possible. Some journals provide a checklist, others leave it up to the contributors to write this section. In the latter case, it is particularly important that all co-authors (or should that be co-contributors?) agree the wording.

One reason why journals are switching to the contributorship system is to prevent **guest** or **ghost authors**. This should not be a problem if you have set up your **writing group** carefully and involved all the **key people/players**. Whether a journal uses a traditional author by-line or a contributor list, those listed should always meet agreed criteria for authorship.

The following references provide some background on the topic.

Horton R (1996) Signing up for authorship. *The Lancet.* **347**: 780.

Rennie D (1997) When authorship fails. A proposal to make contributors accountable. *JAMA.* **278**: 579–85.

Smith R (1997) Authorship: time for a paradigm shift? *BMJ.* **314**: 992.

Wager E (2006) Bye-bye by line, hello contributors. *J Roy Soc Med.* **99**: 1–2

■ Controlled circulation journals; *see* pay journals

■ COPE; *see* Committee on Publication Ethics

■ Copy editing; *see technical editing*

■ Copyright

If you want to reproduce a figure, a table or a large section of text from another publication you need permission from the copyright owner. Until recently, this was nearly always the journal or book publisher. Thus, authors needed permission to reproduce items from their own publications because they did not own the copyright. However, the situation has changed in recent years, and many of the electronic and **Open Access journals** now allow authors to retain copyright on their own work.

Copyright relates to the way in which something appears on paper, i.e. the exact form of wording, or the precise form of a figure. It does not apply to the underlying data. Thus, if you present your data in another form, you will not be breaking copyright. Strictly speaking this means that if you redraw a graph and make some slight alterations to the labelling, you probably do not need permission. However, it is courteous to request permission, and this may prevent later problems. Large publishers have permissions departments that deal with such requests and usually handle them promptly. Some will ask for a fee (although this is rare for non-commercial uses), and most will stipulate the acknowledgement wording you should use.

Short quotations from other academic works do not require permission, but you should clearly indicate that these are quotations and cite the source. Publishers of song lyrics and modern fiction usually guard their copyright fiercely and may deny permission to quote, or charge a substantial fee, so make sure you get permission if you want to use a line from your favourite pop song as a catchy **title**.

Most journals require copies of permission letters on submission, so make your requests as soon as you decide to include copyright material to avoid delays later on.

■ Corrections (errata)

If, despite everybody's best care and attention, you discover an error in something you have published you should contact the journal and ask for a correction to be published. If the journal is indexed on Medline, corrections will be linked to the original article.

If you are feeling pedantic, you can impress the editor by knowing that the term 'correction' should be used for author errors and 'erratum' for the journal's own mistakes. If you want to be old-fashioned you can say 'corrigendum' instead of 'correction' (but they both mean that something has gone wrong).

■ Corresponding author

The corresponding author acts as the point of contact with the journal and will receive the reviewers' comments and proofs. The corresponding author's full contact details, or at least an e-mail address, are usually published with the paper so that readers can contact him/her and request reprints. For other authors, only the affiliation or a short address (e.g. hospital name and city) is usually published.

Since the corresponding author will receive reviewers' comments and proofs, it makes sense to choose the author who is least likely to move and who is most likely to be contactable and able to deal efficiently and rapidly with proofs.

While journals view the corresponding author as a purely administrative designation, some researchers seem to equate this position with the study **guarantor**, or consider it indicates some degree of honour or prestige. It is hard to say whether readers share these views. *See* **order of authors** for more discussion on this tricky subject.

■ Council of Science Editors (CSE)

This was founded in 1957 as the Council of Biology Editors (CBE) and changed its name in 2000 to reflect its broader membership, although it still has a strong biomedical slant. Membership is open to anybody with an interest in science editing; professional North American journal editors and publishers are particularly well represented. CSE holds an annual meeting and occasional retreats, all in North America, and publishes *Science Editor*. The CSE website, www.councilscience editors.org is an excellent resource containing thoughtful statements about a range of issues such as authorship. The meetings are a good way to meet editors, hear their concerns and maybe even buy them a beer.

■ Covering letter (submission letter)

Do not overlook the task of composing a persuasive covering letter in the euphoria of having got everything agreed and the drudgery of sorting out the submission package. This is your chance to 'sell' your submission to the journal editor, but you should remain objective and avoid the 'hard sell'. Start by spelling the editor's name correctly and make sure you are addressing the current incumbent, not a long-deceased predecessor. Then describe your work in a few sentences and explain why you feel it is important. Make the editor's life easier and reap the benefits of careful journal selection by explaining how your work matches the journal's aims and scope, and will be of interest to its readers. If you are aiming at a particular section of the journal, or there is a choice of format (e.g. short or full reports) you should specify this. You should also show that you understand the journal's requirements, for instance by including a statement that the paper has not been published elsewhere and is not being considered by any other journals. Many journals require authors to complete forms about **conflict of interest** but, if not, you should include a statement about this in your letter.

You will also need to write a covering letter when responding to reviewers' comments. Your response should always include a detailed list of the changes you have made and reasons why you have not followed a particular suggestion. This list may form part of your covering letter or may be a separate document.

■ **CSE;** *see* **Council of Science Editors**

D

■ **Data access;** *see* **Access to data**

■ **Data analysis plan**

Statistical analysis is a crucial part of research methodology. Every trial plan, no matter how straightforward, should therefore include a description of how the data will be analysed. This may form part of the trial protocol or a separate data analysis plan. Somebody with statistical expertise should advise on the appropriate methods to use. The plan should set out the primary endpoints of the study and will often include a power calculation to indicate the sample size needed to confirm or refute the underlying hypothesis with confidence. Whatever the **key message(s)** of the publication, it is important to distinguish primary endpoints from secondary or *post hoc* analyses. The data analysis plan should help to ensure that a study is analysed and reported responsibly. A medical writer preparing a draft should have access to the plan to determine the primary endpoints and for details such as power calculations and randomisation methods which are required to fulfil the **CONSORT** requirements.

Developing the initial publication strategy and the data analysis plan at the same time can save a lot of time and trouble later. For example, if you consider what tables you might include in a publication you can ensure that the analysis will provide these.

■ **Data dredging**

This disparaging term refers to the practice of analysing data well beyond any reasonable scientific or statistical bounds in a desperate search for significant-looking p-values or the hope of wringing out some publication-worthy droplets. It therefore tends to result in **redundant publications**, or even to completely fallacious ones. The simple rule to avoid data dredging is to have a **data analysis plan** and stick to it. Occasionally, *post hoc* analyses will be justified if you notice interesting patterns in your data or want to explore a new hypothesis, but always seek the advice of a statistician about the validity of such analyses and, if you do try to publish them, make sure secondary analyses are clearly labelled as such and that appropriate statistical methods have been used to correct for multiple analyses.

■ Data ownership; *see* ownership of data

■ DataVision

Web-based publication planning software developed by Envision Pharma. It provides project management tools and databases giving information about journals and congresses. *See* www.envisionpharma.com for details.

■ Deadlines

Meetings usually have strict deadlines for **abstract** submission. Occasionally, exceptions can be made and abstracts accepted after the deadline, but do not count on this. Generally, the larger the meeting, the firmer the deadline. If you know your results will only be available a few days after the deadline it might be worth contacting the meeting organisers and asking if they can extend the deadline or if **late breaker abstracts** will be accepted. Try to do this as far in advance as possible. Submission deadlines sometimes get extended if the organisers receive fewer abstracts than they had hoped for – but again, you should not count on this, even if it has happened in previous years.

The only deadline you are likely to encounter from a journal is one for returning proofs. After waiting several months for these to arrive, this can sometimes be unexpectedly short, e.g. 48 hours. Failure to return corrected proofs within this deadline may delay publication until the next issue. This is why it makes sense to inform the journal if the **corresponding author**'s contact details change, and to nominate somebody for this role who is likely to respond quickly.

■ Decision times

Although electronic submission and reviewing may have trimmed a few days off journal schedules, external reviewers remain the rate-limiting step in the peer-review process. Most journals do not pay their reviewers (or offer only a nominal reward) so editors cannot demand a rapid response. Good reviewers are also hard to find, so editors are keen not to antagonise or overburden them. Because of this, authors often have to wait several weeks, and sometimes several months, for a decision from traditional journals. (The median time from submission to acceptance for *JAMA* in 2008 was 56 days but that represents a considerable improvement from the 103 day average in 2004.) However, in journals that use in-house review to screen all submissions, average times for rejection may be much shorter than those for acceptance. (The median time from receipt to rejection at *JAMA* in 2008 was eight days.)

Aware of the frustration caused by waiting for decisions, and also of the fact that drug companies may be prepared to pay for a more rapid service, some pay journals offer rapid review for all submissions. For example, *Current Medical Research & Opinion* takes, on average, 14 days for a provisional acceptance or rejection.

Other journals that don't normally impose page charges offer rapid review for a fee. For example, the *International Journal of Clinical Practice* (which usually reckons to take about 20 days for peer review and to produce proofs about 10 days after acceptance) offers an expedited review service that ensures peer review within seven days of online submission and proofs within seven days of acceptance. However, expedited review is only available for clinical trials (which must conform with the **CONSORT** or STROBE reporting guidelines).

Do not confuse journals that offer quick decisions for all or some papers with the practice of having a **fast-track publication** route for papers of exceptional interest. Remember that the editor will decide whether your paper merits special treatment and, by definition, this is only going to apply to a few, remarkable studies. If speed of publication is important, it is better to select your target journal carefully than to rely on rapid review in a big-name journal.

See also **acceptance times** and **rejection times** and Chapter 3 'How long will it take?' (pp. 13–16) for more details.

■ DOI (Digital Object Identifier) system

The DOI system was introduced to overcome some of the difficulties of citing electronic material. It is administered by the International DOI Foundation, which defines a DOI as 'a persistent identifier of intellectual property entities'. Some journals now assign DOIs to every article. They act like a postcode and could, in theory, replace traditional citations, but since they are long, unmemorable strings of numbers and letters, this seems unlikely unless human intelligence evolves unexpectedly. DOIs are especially useful for citing electronic references, **supplementary material**, or items posted on a journal's website before the print edition, which have not yet had volume or page numbers assigned. The system also forms the basis for CrossRef, a not-for-profit initiative that allows publishers to cross-link citations so readers can go directly from an article to a cited reference in a few mouse clicks.

For more information go to http://www.doi.org or http://www.crossref.org

■ Duplicate publication; *see* redundant publication

E

■ EASE; *see* European Association of Science Editors

■ Economic (health outcomes) evaluations

These are often published as secondary papers (i.e. separately from the original clinical trial results) in specialist health economics journals. However, such journals tend to be read by economists rather than by prescribers. Some editors consider that economic aspects can only be evaluated in the context of clinical findings and, for this reason, the *BMJ* will not accept economic evaluations without the clinical results.[1] Introduced in 2002, this policy does not seem to have been adopted by other journals or incorporated in the **International Committee of Medical Journal Editors' (ICMJE)** 'Uniform Requirements . . .', but it is worth checking instructions carefully in case your target journal has a similar policy.

1 Smith R (2002) New *BMJ* policy on economic evaluations. *BMJ.* **325**: 1124.

■ Editorial board

Most journals have editorial boards but their composition and role vary greatly. Having a contact on the editorial board might be an advantage, but in order to appreciate just how much (or how little) influence this person may have, you need to understand the board's role in a particular journal. Editorial board members are usually listed on the journal website or inside the front cover. The first thing to do is count them. If your chum is one of dozens, then his/her influence is likely to be limited. If, on the other hand, there are fewer than 12 members, you might really have a friend at court. Next look at the journal's instructions to contributors. If members of the editorial board are assigned to handle certain papers, then this suggests they may perform an important screening function and may act, in effect, as the editor for their region or subject area. Finally, try to find out if and when the editorial board meets. The strongest clue to this is given in journals that publish acceptance dates for papers: if the papers published in each issue seem to have been accepted on only one or two dates, this suggests an active editorial board that meets to decide what to accept. In contrast, some journals use their editorial board mainly as a figurehead in which case it will meet only rarely and its members are virtually never used as reviewers – let alone expected to discuss the fate of papers. In this case, it may do no harm to contact your friend to ask his or her general advice about whether your paper is suited to the journal, but you cannot expect much more. In the worst case, board members may be dead (making them especially hard to contact and unlikely to intercede on your behalf).

See **review process** for more details about how journals organise their peer review.

■ Editorials

In many journals, editorials or commentaries accompany research papers or comment on important developments. Such 'opinion pieces' are usually commissioned by the journal, often from somebody who reviewed the paper or who is an expert in the field. In *The Lancet*, the editorials are always written by a member of staff and appear under the **by-line** 'Lancet'. However the journal also publishes commentaries. If you have an idea for an editorial or commentary it is best to contact the editor informally to discover whether the journal considers uncommissioned pieces, and, if so, whether it might be interested in yours. Editorials to accompany an article may have to be prepared quickly so as not to delay publication.

The purpose of editorials and commentaries is to present the commentator's views on the meaning of a publication or the implications of a new policy or development. They usually contain a few references but can include more unsubstantiated opinion than other types of publication.

Since they express an opinion, it is important that the writer's voice is heard, and it is usually inappropriate for another party to suggest what the author should write or how they should tackle the subject. For this reason, the first version of the **Good Publication Practice (GPP)** guidelines for pharmaceutical companies recommended that, while it is acceptable for a professional writer or editor to polish an editorial for an author (e.g. to help a non-native English speaker) it is not usually acceptable for anybody other than the named author to prepare the first draft.

■ Editors

There are several types of editor and it is important to understand their different roles. The Editor (or Editor-in-Chief) of a journal is the overall boss, having the final decision over what gets published and responsibility for setting the journal's policies. He or she may be advised and assisted by committees, editorial boards and junior editors, but, the Editor (with a capital 'E') carries final responsibility. Editors may be full-time professionals employed by the journal (or its parent organisation) or part-timers doing their editing job on top of another. Full-time Editors usually work from a journal or publishers office, while part-time ones usually work from their own institution. The level of administrative support available to different types of editors therefore varies. If you contact a secretary or assistant in a journal office it is reasonable to expect that s/he is familiar with the journal's processes and may have access to files. On the other hand, a secretary in a university or hospital may have virtually nothing to do with her boss' editorial responsibilities.

Working alongside the Editor may be assistant editors with responsibility for sections of the journal (e.g. correspondence) or a proportion of submissions. Finally, there is another species of editor responsible for preparing accepted typescripts for printing. These are called technical editors, desk editors or sub-editors depending on the journal. This type of editor takes no part in deciding what gets published but will put submissions into **house style** and check proofs (*see* **technical editing** for more details). If you find major problems in the proofs, it is usually best to discuss them directly with the sub-editor who prepared the manuscript. In the case of journals edited by part-time editors, technical editing may be done by somebody employed (or hired) by the academic society or publisher, or by the Editor. Check the contact details supplied with the proofs to determine the best person to contact.

To complete the classification, we should not forget authors' editors who help authors prepare submissions. They may be employed by the authors' institution (especially in the case of large US universities) or may be freelance.

■ Electronic publishing

Many journals that started life, and are still firmly rooted, in traditional paper and print use the internet or electronic media to some extent. They have been joined by wholly electronic publications that exist solely on the internet or are distributed in electronic form, for example as CD-ROMs. The term 'electronic publishing' seems to cover all aspects of this wide spectrum, making it, unless clearly defined, rather meaningless.

However, when choosing a journal you should consider how it is published, since this will affect not only the speed of publication but also the journal's accessibility and how it is likely to be perceived. Medical journals fall into two broad categories – those that are purely electronic, such as the **BioMed Central** and **Public Library of Science (PLoS)** journals, and those that still use print as the version of record but offer various electronic functions, such as *The Lancet*. A few, such as the *BMJ*, are true hybrids, offering longer versions of papers on the website and extra features such as rapid responses. If you have very large data tables, or want to include media such as video clips, it is worth considering journals that can publish **supplementary material** electronically.

Since purely electronic journals are not constrained by production and distribution costs (and therefore do not have to work within a page budget) they often have higher acceptance rates than print journals. Electronic journals also tend to have a considerably shorter **lead time** from acceptance to publication since articles do not have to wait for the next printed issue. On the negative side, electronic journals tend to invest less in **technical editing** than printed ones, and, being newer and easier to get into are generally considered less prestigious. Until recently, electronic journals were not assigned **impact factors** (which was a major drawback for some potential academic authors), but this situation has now been rectified.

As well as traditional journal metrics, some electronic journals now offer article-level metrics so you can see how many people have downloaded or cited your work (the PLoS system is explained at http://article-level-metrics.plos.org). Some journals also encourage readers to rate, annotate or comment on articles which could be great if they say nice things about your research but not so welcome if they are critical.

Other benefits are that most are **Open Access journals**, or are available via

PubMed Central, reducing the importance of indexing.

Although not strictly related to their electronic status, some of the newer journals practise open (unblinded) peer review, and some take this one stage further by making reviewers' comments available to readers.

■ Electronic review

Most journals use e-mail to communicate with reviewers. Although this has several advantages, and should, in theory, shorten review time, it probably has not accelerated the process enormously, as the rate-limiting step remains the busy (and unpaid) reviewer. If the reviewer reads the paper on screen it might even save a few trees – but I bet most reviewers still print submissions out.

On a less curmudgeonly note, electronic review does offer potential advantages, such as automatic links to references cited in the submission, or to guidelines for reviewers. It also enables potential reviewers to read an **abstract** before deciding whether to accept the invitation to review – this might help to identify competing interests earlier, although a study at *Annals of Emergency Medicine* suggested that it does not speed up the review process.

■ Electronic submission

Most journals permit or even mandate electronic submission of articles. This may slightly reduce the workload of preparing the submission package, since it generally takes less time to make an electronic submission than to prepare three, four or even five copies of your paper and post them. Check the instructions to contributors for details of file formats, etc. that are acceptable. Formatting details that often cause problems (and which journals therefore often ask you to remove) include fixed page breaks, right-hand justification and tables aligned using spaces rather than tabs or table settings. Special characters such as Greek letters or accents often get lost in transmission. It is therefore safer to use alternatives such as mcg for micrograms (rather than µg) or spelling out alpha and beta. Pay careful attention to special characters when you paste text into a form for submitting an abstract to a conference – I have seen very odd things happen to Greek characters and symbols, such as less than (<).

Even if you submit a paper or abstract electronically, you may still have to send hard copies of signed forms such as copyright transfers or authorship statements.

Many conferences now send automatic acknowledgements of electronically submitted abstracts, which is reassuring. However, as with any submission, you should make a note when you do it and contact the journal or meeting if you have received no acknowledgement after about a month. Both paper and electronic submissions do sometimes get lost in transmission/the post, or at the editorial office, so it is reasonable to expect some sort of acknowledgement.

■ ELPS

This acronym is used by the *BMJ* to stand for Electronic Long, Paper Short[1] referring to the fact that articles in the printed version are shorter than those on the website. Although most journals do not go as far as the *BMJ* (which invests heavily in editors who trim the paper version) many with websites will post **supplementary material**, such as large data tables, copies of questionnaires, or video clips, which cannot be accommodated in the printed version.

If you have a lot of data to present, or want to use an unconventional medium (such as video), study the journal's website, check the instructions to authors, or contact the editorial office to see if they can handle this.

1 *See* Mullner M and Groves T (2002) Making research papers in the *BMJ* more accessible. *BMJ*. **325**: 456 and Schroter S, Barratt H and Smith J (2004) Authors' perceptions of electronic publishing: two cross-sectional surveys. *BMJ*. **328**: 1350–3.

■ Envision

Commercial company that provides **DataVision** publication planning tools

■ EQUATOR Network

An international initiative to improve the reporting of medical research. EQUATOR stands for Enhancing the QUAlity and Transparency Of health Research. It was started by members of the team that developed **CONSORT**, but their resource centre gives useful links to a wide range of guidelines so this website is a good place to check if there are any guidelines on the type of research you are trying to publish.

www.equator-network.org

■ Errata; *see* corrections

■ European Association of Science Editors (EASE)

This was founded in 1982 from the merger of the European Life Sciences Editors Association and Editerra, an association for earth science editors. Membership is not restricted to Europe, and EASE currently has members from over 50 countries.

EASE holds meetings every three years. Unlike **WAME** and **CSE**, EASE has not issued statements on editorial policy, but it has produced a handbook for editors. It publishes *European Science Editing* which includes peer-reviewed research articles as well as association news and useful summaries of papers about all aspects of editing and publishing. Membership of EASE includes academic (i.e. part-time) editors, technical editors and translators, as well as professional editors and publishers.

For more information look at www.ease.org.uk

■ European Medical Writers Association (EMWA)

As the name suggests, this is an organisation for medical writers. It developed from the American Medical Writers Association (AMWA) in 1989 and now largely functions independently. EMWA has produced guidelines on the role of professional medical writers in developing publications (*see* Appendix 3, pp. 139–45). These guidelines aim to reduce the problems associated with ghost writers.

For details visit www.emwa.org

Jacobs A and Wager E (2005) EMWA guidelines on the role of medical writers in developing peer-reviewed publications. *Curr Med Res Opin.* **21**(2): 317–21.

■ Expectations

A publication is usually the end-product of a collaboration involving many people. Devising, agreeing and communicating a successful publication strategy therefore depends on discovering the expectations of everybody involved. Depending on their background, previous experience and personality, people can have widely different expectations. Do not assume that you know what individuals hope to get out of a publication, or what they expect the processes will be.

The relationship between research sponsors and investigators can be a complex and delicate one. Involvement of extra parties such as contract research organisations (CROs), communications agencies or freelance professional writers can add further layers of complexity. The first step in establishing expectations is to make sure that all **key players** have been consulted and offered the chance to contribute. For large studies, this is likely to involve a wider group than just the named authors.

The best way to find out what people expect is to arrange a **meeting** involving as many key players as possible. If this is difficult, then a telephone or video conference is probably the next best thing. Appoint somebody to chair the meeting or lead the phone conference, and somebody else to record the decisions.

When discussing a publication strategy try to cover all the issues. The most important ones to establish are:

- timing
- target meetings (for abstracts)
- target journal (for primary publication)
- number of publications
- authorship
- key messages

- roles (i.e. who does what).

When these are agreed, write them down and circulate the information. Memories are unreliable, and written notes will also help to inform those who could not take part in the discussion.

If circumstances change, keep checking expectations and consulting the key players. Always consider if you have left anybody out (e.g. an investigator who might expect to be an author). If in doubt, increase your communication network rather than narrowing it. Differences in expectations are best settled well before crucial deadlines (e.g. for abstract submission) and at the earliest stages of publication development.

The best way of checking expectations on a full paper is to circulate an **outline** for comment before preparing a first draft. It is far better to uncover differences in interpretation and emphasis at this stage than when you are just about to submit the paper.

Many publishing conventions are unwritten. I have been mystified by authors squabbling over who should be named as the **corresponding author**, or why they like the convention that male authors are listed with their initials, but female authors have their forenames spelled out in full. Even experienced researchers can have strange misconceptions about publication processes, and everybody has their own idiosyncrasies, prejudices and opinions. The only method to guarantee a smooth process is to make no assumptions, discover everybody's expectations about what should happen, and keep the lines of communication open.

■ Expedited review

A posh term for a fast-track review system which some journals offer for a fee. *See* **decision times** for more details.

■ External review

The traditional model of peer review, and probably the one that most authors expect journals to use, involves sending papers to external reviewers (i.e. independent experts who are not employed by the journal). However, journals that employ a large editorial team reject a considerable proportion of submissions without external review. Such journals (which tend to be the large, general weekly journals such as *The Lancet* and *NEJM*) always use external reviewers before papers are accepted, but they reject as many as 30–50% of submissions on internal review. The advantage of internal screening (or **in-house review**) is that it usually produces a rapid decision. The disadvantage is that authors receive a less detailed critique – often just a letter stating that the submission is not suitable for the journal.

F

■ Fast-track publication

Some journals offer rapid publication (within about four weeks of acceptance) for papers that represent major breakthroughs or have important public health implications. However, apart from a few journals that offer ultra-speedy publication if you pay an extra fee, you cannot generally demand a place on the fast-track just because it is convenient for you. The decision to accept a paper as fast-track rests with the editor. Few papers are deemed worthy of fast-tracking, for example *The Lancet* accepts about 50 per year. You will therefore need to construct a very persuasive **covering letter** to explain exactly why your paper merits special attention. *The Lancet*'s instructions to contributors recommend calling the editor for a preliminary discussion. Since the advent of **electronic publishing**, some journals now post important papers on their website before print publication.

Since only a handful of exceptional papers will be afforded this honour, you should not expect fast-track as a right. After you have devoted years of your life to a piece of research you are bound to believe it is of enormous importance. Try to take a step back or get your most sceptical colleagues' views before assuming that your paper will qualify. Very few individual studies answer an important question so clearly that they change the practice of medicine. Mostly, science evolves gradually and your research will represent one piece of a larger jigsaw. If speed of publication is vital, it is better to choose your target journal carefully than to rely on fast-track review in a major journal. Some electronic journals and **pay journals** routinely offer rapid decisions and minimal **lead time** from acceptance to publication, and, as these journals generally have higher acceptance rates than traditional print journals, this is undoubtedly a more reliable route to guarantee prompt publication.

The conference equivalent of the journal's fast-track is **late breaker abstracts**.

Goldbeck-Wood S (1999) *BMJ* introduces a fast track system for papers. *BMJ.* **318**: 620, but see also an alternative view, Martyn C (2005) Slow tracking for *BMJ* papers. *BMJ.* **331:** 1551–2.

■ FDAAA

This rather unpronounceable acronym stands for the equally unwieldy Food and Drug Administration Amendments Act of 2007, which despite its date (which refers to when it was passed), comes into force from 2008 to 2010. The Act requires tabular summaries of the results of most Phase II to IV studies to be posted on **ClinicalTrials. gov** within 12 months of the study ending. In response to this, many drug companies now try to publish a full paper in a journal by about the same time as the results summary is posted, to provide context and interpretation to complement the very dry summary tables. This can set tough deadlines for publication planners who therefore do not have time to say 'FDA Amendments Act' and refer to it as 'Fe-daah'.

Wager E (2008) FDAAA Legislation: Global Implications for Clinical Trial Reporting and Publication Planning. Keyword Pharma Report 2008. http://www.keywordpharma.com/prods/wager3.asp

■ Fees; *see* page charges; pay journals

■ Figure legends

Requirements for these may vary with electronic submission but many journals still expect figure legends (headings) to be listed all together at the end of the document rather than with each figure. This reflects the old printing technology in which words were typeset along with the text while figures had to be processed and inserted separately. Even if your software allows you to insert figures into a document, many journals require you to submit them as separate files, with the legends listed after the text.

Aim to make figure legends comprehensible to someone who has only scanned the text, for example by spelling out abbreviations. References in legends can cause problems, especially if the journal uses the Vancouver (sequential numbering) system, since you cannot tell exactly where the figure will appear in the text until the pages are made up. It is therefore helpful to refer to the author and date, as well as giving a number. If a figure is taken from another work you must obtain **permission** from the copyright holder (*see* **copyright**) and it is usual to mention this in the legend. If a figure has been adapted from another source it is courteous to acknowledge this even though you may not require formal permission. Typical wording would be:

> Fig. X. The renin-angiotensin system (reproduced from Baggins *et al.*[Ref c] by permission of Journals-R-Us Inc.).

■ Figures

The familiar equation that 'a picture is worth a thousand words' does not necessarily hold in scientific publishing. The 'rules' governing figures are often unwritten, and are definitely different for posters and papers.

Posters at conferences tend to be skimmed rapidly, rather than read, so the aim is to get your message across quickly and clearly. Figures such as flow diagrams, bar charts and pie charts are effective ways to display study designs and results, and should be used freely. If space permits, you can even show data both in a table and a graph (a luxury not permitted in a paper). Use your judgement to choose between including a lot of detail, and presenting clean, clear graphics. Some details, such as error bars, may be essential for understanding the data, others, such as exact patient numbers for every parameter measured, may be unnecessary. Pie charts and stacked bars are good for showing differences in proportions. Bar charts are good for comparing pairs of data, such as mean values from different treatment groups. Line graphs are good for showing changes over time. Use colours consistently (e.g. to indicate different treatment groups) and avoid red/green contrasts since about one in 12 men have some degree of colour-blindness and cannot distinguish these colours.

Journals often impose restrictions on the number and type of figures you can include in a paper. The general rule is that you must not duplicate information between text, tables and figures. You must therefore choose the best form for presenting your data. Unlike posters, papers are usually considered the 'publication of record', in other words, the definitive and lasting report of a piece of research. Papers may be used for systematic reviews or meta-analyses which require considerable detail. For these reasons (and, perhaps because, in the past, typesetting and reproducing figures cost more than printing text or tables) journal editors usually favour tables over figures.

A simple bar chart comparing values from two groups is unlikely to be accepted in a paper. It is usually best to present this sort of data in a table, which allows you to show the actual values, a measure of the dispersion (e.g. standard deviation) and statistical significance (e.g. 95% confidence interval or p-value).

However, other kinds of figures, such as those that synthesise a lot of data points, are usually acceptable, for example scatter plots or regression analyses and survival curves (e.g. Kaplan-Meier plots). Line graphs showing changes over several time points can also be useful if they complement the text or table rather than duplicate it.

Images such as X-rays, CT-scans or photomicrographs can be useful in case reports or to illustrate an unusual finding within a study. Photographs of patients may also be useful, but should be included only if you have obtained specific consent from the subject. It is not acceptable simply to blank out the eyes in an attempt to anonymise an image. Some journals require evidence of patient consent for publication. Make sure that images such as CT- and ultrasound scans do not contain details that might identify the subject.

If you want to reproduce a figure from another publication (even one of your own) you must obtain permission from the **copyright** owner (usually the publisher, but see the section on **permissions** for details). Many journals require evidence that permission has been obtained, so sort this out in good time before you plan to submit.

When preparing a paper, figures are always presented separately, at the end (for print copies) or in a separate file (for electronic). Even though your word processor will allow you to embed figures in the text, you should not do so. Some journals also require figure legends to be submitted separately from the figures. (This convention dates back to old printing technology in which text was typeset separately and figures were then slotted into the pages. Although this is now obsolete, some journals still request it, and obeying their request shows that you have, at least, read their instructions which will, no doubt, please the old-fashioned editors who still require it.)

Most journals do not use colour printing for papers, and those that do (e.g. *The Lancet* has gone technicolour) will convert your figures into their colour scheme. Graphics should therefore be prepared in black and white. Some journals charge to include colour photographs – check the instructions for details.

Many software packages such as Excel and Lotus allow you to prepare simple figures. However, if you want to add error bars or use more sophisticated graphics you will need specialist software. Remember that figures are usually produced larger than they will appear in print, so labels, in particular, must survive reduction. The default settings for label size on programs such as Excel or PowerPoint are designed for printing on A4 (or 8″ × 11″) paper or preparing slides, so they are usually too small.

Before spending a lot of time preparing your own graphs, check the formats acceptable to the journal. It may save a lot of time to get graphs drawn by a professional illustrator who can supply formats such as .eps files which can be submitted electronically to journals, or high quality glossy prints suitable for printing.

If you are planning a budget for getting a paper published, remember to include the cost of preparing figures and for copyright charges (if you want to reproduce published figures). It may often be quicker and cheaper, and the results certainly more appealing, to get figures professionally drawn than to expect investigators or writers to produce them.

■ First author; *see* order of authors

■ Footnotes

Most medical journals do not allow footnotes. The only exception is that some journals use footnotes to acknowledge funding or to list study group members who are not identified individually on the by-line. (However, do not assume that listing names in a footnote means that these individuals do not need to fulfil authorship criteria – *see* **by-lines**, **order of authors** and **contributorship vs. authorship** for more details on this tricky area.)

Another possible exception is if new data emerge after a paper is typeset and you want to add an update to the proofs. Rather than re-setting large sections of text, or renumbering references, the journal might prefer this to appear as a footnote – although, in these days of computer typesetting, this is probably needlessly old-fashioned.

Journals of law or medical ethics, on the other hand, may positively encourage footnotes. The rule, as always, is to check a recent copy of your target journal. If footnotes are permitted, check how these should be included in a manuscript or electronic submission.

Some people use the 'Endnote' function of Word to produce reference lists, although I find dedicated bibliographic software far more efficient. If you have used either of these, check that this does not mess up an electronic submission.

■ Formats

Always check your target journal to see what types of articles it accepts. It is a surprisingly common mistake to identify a journal by its readership or impact factor and to ignore the fact that it simply never publishes the type of paper you have prepared.

Even if a journal publishes the type of article you have in mind, check whether it considers unsolicited manuscripts. Many journals publish only commissioned **editorials** and opinion pieces, so unsolicited ones can be hard to place. Others will not consider unsolicited review articles. The best strategy is to make an initial enquiry to the editor to see if you can interest him/her in your idea.

A few journals will not consider editorials or non-systematic reviews from authors with competing interests. Other, and to my mind more enlightened, journals regard transparency as the key and try to ensure that any potential **conflict of interest** is stated so that reviewers and readers can decide for themselves. Honesty is definitely the best policy – all authors should be prepared to disclose potential competing interests both financial and personal – but bear in mind that this might bar you from publishing certain types of articles in some journals.

■ Freebies / 'throwaways'

Freebies (or 'throwaways') are medical newspapers such as *GP* and *Pulse* in the UK, and *Family Practice News* in the US. They are funded by advertising, sent to large numbers of doctors and quite widely read. They often contain short, practical review or educational articles as well as news items but they virtually never carry original research and rarely accept unsolicited items. If you want to write for the freebies you should contact the editor directly with your ideas, but you should not plan to publish your research this way. However, if your findings are truly earth shattering, or you want to publicise an event or initiative, you might consider issuing a press release in the hope that it will be used in a news item.

G

■ Galley proofs

Strictly speaking, a galley proof is the initial proof stage when text is set to the correct line width but not made up into pages. On a galley proof the text appears as a single, uninterrupted column and the figures and tables do not appear in their final positions. Electronic typesetting has made this stage almost redundant. In most cases, authors receive page proofs, which have the text laid out into the journal's usual page format with tables and figures in their correct places.

These days, the only items that sometimes appear as galley proofs are letters. This is because correspondence is usually squeezed into journals at the last minute, so the number of letters that appear in each issue will depend on how much space the articles occupy. Journal editors may therefore get authors to approve galley proofs of letters and then make up the journal pages when the rest of the issue is finalised.

As letters rarely contain figures or tables, and are often short, this usually poses no problems, so you can treat them like page proofs.

For some reason, some people continue to refer to all proofs as galley proofs (or, to show how well they think they know the jargon, simply as 'galleys'). So that you do not fall into this trap (and as I'm feeling pedantic), you will find details about handling proofs under 'P' for **proofs** (**page proofs**). Incidentally, as I'm being pedantic, you might like to know that the word galley refers to the rectangular tray into which metal type used to be set, not an ancient ship.

■ Ghost author(s)

A ghost author is somebody who qualifies for authorship but is not included in a publication's author list. The occurrence of ghosts is bad for everybody concerned. It deprives the ghost author of recognition and it misleads readers about who did the work. The most common cause of ghosts is sponsors trying to underplay their involvement in studies by limiting the number of company authors, but authors may also be omitted because of professional (academic) rivalry.

The best way to avoid ghost authors is to agree authorship criteria early in the research process. When the study is complete, the criteria should be checked to make sure that everybody who qualifies is included in preparing the publication(s).

Ghost authorship should not be confused with ghost writing – a term sometimes used when a medical writer, who does not qualify for authorship, assists with a publication but it is not acknowledged – read on for further details.

A study of ghost authorship, which looked for people who were named on a study protocol but not on the publication, found that statisticians suffered this spectral fate more often than medical writers.

Gøtzsche PC, Hróbjartsson A, Johansen HK *et al.* (2007) Ghost authorship in industry-initiated randomised trials. *PLoS Med.* 4:e19.

■ Ghost writers

This term is sometimes applied to a professional medical writer who has not been involved with a study but who helps develop a publication – in particular, by preparing the first draft. The term is unfortunate as it implies that the writer's identity is not revealed. However, getting help from a professional writer is no more shameful than getting advice from a professional statistician and the involvement of a writer should not be confused with questions about competing interests or of sponsors trying to exert undue influence over publications. It is therefore important that the writer and their source of funding should be identified (usually in the **acknowledgements** section) which effectively exorcises the paper.

The question of whether a writer qualifies as an author is a matter for judgement. Unless a writer has contributed to the interpretation of the data and is prepared to take public responsibility for the research (not just responsibility for how the publication was prepared) they will not meet the **International Committee of Medical**

Journal Editors' **(ICMJE)** authorship criteria and therefore, in most journals, they should not appear on the **by-line**. However, a few journals (e.g. *Neurology*) argue that the preparation of a draft is, in itself, an act of interpretation, and prefer the writer to be listed as an author, or at least as a contributor (*see* **Acknowledgements**).

How much data interpretation the writer does will depend on how the paper is developed. Both **Good Publication Practice (GPP)** for pharmaceutical companies and the **EMWA** guidelines recommend that a draft should not be prepared until an **outline** has been agreed with the named authors. If a detailed outline and **key messages** are established from discussions with the named authors, the writer may have only a limited role in deciding how data are presented or interpreted. However, if a writer takes a more active role, for example by searching and synthesising the literature for a review article or for the introduction or discussion sections of a primary paper, then the writer's contribution may merit authorship.

The EMWA guidelines for medical writers and GPP for pharmaceutical companies contain practical recommendations for the appropriate use of medical writers in developing publications. *See* Appendix 3 (pp. 139–66) where both the guidelines can be studied in detail.

See also Chapter 4 'Working with a medical writer'.

■ Gift authorship; *see* guest authors

■ Good Publication Practice (GPP and GPP2)

This is a set of guidelines developed by people within the pharmaceutical industry to encourage the responsible and ethical development of publications. Although the guidelines refer to both the **International Committee of Medical Journal Editors'** **(ICMJE)** 'Uniform Requirements . . .' and the **CONSORT** Statement, they go beyond both of these, in particular by including detailed recommendations about the role of professional medical writers – something about which most other guidelines are silent.

The original GPP guidelines arose from a meeting in 1999 between journal editors, academic investigators and drug company personnel. One area of particular concern for both the editors and the academics was **publication bias**, i.e. the tendency for favourable findings to be published more than negative ones. GPP therefore called on companies to endeavour to publish the results of all clinical trials of marketed products. GPP also provided guidance on ways to avoid covert **redundant publication**, such as clear study identification. The first version of GPP was published in 2003.

GPP was endorsed by several drug companies, supported by a number of communication agencies, and included in the instructions to contributors of the *BMJ* and **BioMed Central** journals.

For more details *see* www.gpp-guidelines.org

The GPP guidelines have been revised after extensive consultation coordinated by ISMPP, resulting in the publication of GPP2 in late 2009.

See Appendix 3 (pp. 139–66) where the guidelines are reproduced.

Wager E, Field EA and Grossman L (2003) Good Publication Practice for pharmaceutical companies. *Curr Med Res Opin.* **19**: 149–54.

Graf C, Battisti WP, Bridges D *et al* (2009) Good Publication Practice for communicating company sponsored medical research. *BMJ.* **339**: b4330.

■ Graphs

See also **figures**. If you use graphs a lot, and enjoy fiddling about with this sort of thing, then it may be worth investing in specialist software to produce them. However, although such packages are versatile and powerful, they take a while to learn and it is easy to forget what all the features do unless you use them frequently. I therefore find it easier, quicker (and, if you are counting your time, cheaper) to get graphs prepared by a professional illustrator or designer. Such people can produce high quality figures in formats acceptable to journals.

■ Group authorship

Authorship by a group (rather than a list of individuals) is sometimes suggested, perhaps in the hope of avoiding difficult decisions about author order and number. Although this may seem like a neat solution, it has some drawbacks. For a start, some journals won't allow it, so check your target journal. Secondly, databases such as Medline often don't handle group names very cleverly, so they may be mis-cited. There is even evidence that studies with only group authors are cited less often than those with real people on the by-line.[1]

Acknowledging a group in addition to individuals is generally a better idea, but you still need to check your target journal. Some journals will allow Author N, Writer A on behalf of the CHUMMY Study Group and will print a list of members of the study group. Others insist that all listed group members meet authorship criteria – which rather defeats the object. Medline permits collaborators to be listed and recognises these are different from authors. It notes that 'When a group name for a specific consortium, committee, study group, or the like appears in an article byline, the personal names of the members of that group may be published in the article text. Such names are entered as collaborator names for the Medline citation. Collaborator names are entered . . . only when a group (corporate) author name is present'.
www.nlm.nih.gov/pubs/factsheets/authorship.html

1 Dickersin K, Scherer R, Suci ES *et al.* (2002) Problems with indexing and citation of articles with group authorship. *JAMA.* **287**: 2772–4.

■ Guarantor

Journals that have adopted the **contributorship** system (i.e. those that list individuals' contributions to a piece of work) may ask that one contributor guarantees the project's integrity. The idea behind this is that individuals may have specialist roles within complex studies. It is therefore unreasonable to expect the statistician to justify the choice of dose, or for a clinician to explain why a certain statistical test was used. However, if each person takes responsibility for only part of the study somebody needs to act as a guarantor for the overall project. Check your target journal's instructions (or a recent issue) to see if you need to nominate a guarantor. Conventionally, this person will often be the first or **last author**, but there are no rules about this.

■ Guest authors / gift authorship

Guests are people who are invited to be listed as authors although they do not meet authorship criteria (or fulfil the criteria less well than others who are not included). Guests are usually included for their prestige, in the hope that adding their name will increase a publication's chances of acceptance or its impact on readers. They may also be included to curry favour or for mutual CV enlargement. The latter occurs in competitive academic fields, or those in which promotion or tenure depends on the length (rather than the quality) of a person's publication list, when researchers add colleagues' names to papers on the understanding that the colleagues will do the same for them. Drug companies may be tempted to offer guest authorship to eminent opinion leaders in the hope that this will endear them to the company and add credibility to the research, although, if the practice is disclosed, it could have the opposite effect.

Whatever the motive, guest authorship should be discouraged, since it presents a dishonest picture of how a study was performed, is likely to irritate the 'real' authors, and may increase the likelihood of deserving authors being omitted.

However, the habit may be hard to break if there is a strong tradition of the professor being included in every publication from his or her department. It is a brave junior researcher who is prepared to question this practice even armed with clear guidance from the target journal and the **International Committee of Medical Journal Editors' (ICMJE)** criteria, which state that obtaining funding or general supervision of a research group, by themselves, are not automatic qualifications for authorship. The moves by journals toward listing individuals' contributions rather than just their names (i.e. **contributorship**) may help discourage guest authorship, since it may help readers and editors to identify guests. However, with the traditional author **by-line** it is usually impossible for anybody outside the research team to distinguish deserving authors from guests. Some journals require authors to sign a statement that they meet the ICMJE criteria; however, people prepared to accept gift authorship are often quite happy to make a dishonest declaration so this probably has little effect.

Institutional authorship policies, in particular outlawing the practice of always including the head of department, are likely to be more effective. But, sadly, few academic institutions have such policies in place. Junior researchers seeking ammunition may find the COPE guidelines on authorship (available at www.publication ethics.org) helpful – but I am probably biased, as I am one of the authors (and not a guest).

H

■ Hanging Committee

This is the name of a *BMJ* committee that used to be the final judge of whether submissions were accepted. It got its name from the committee at London's Royal Academy that selects pictures to hang on the walls at its summer exhibition (although to rejected authors its actions may have resembled capital punishment).

In other journals the **editorial board** may serve a similar function. At *The Lancet*, papers are discussed by all editors at a weekly meeting (but it doesn't have a funny name).

■ Hot topics

Journal acceptance rates are, by definition, averages. One way of increasing your chance of acceptance is by researching your **target journal** well. This means not only knowing the types of articles it publishes, but reading the most recent issues to see if any themes or 'hot topics' emerge. Unfortunately, you can't usually plan your research to coincide with a journal editor's latest interest; however, given a choice; of two rather similar journals, only one of which has published papers on a similar theme to yours, it is a good idea to select that journal.

However, you should not confuse hot topics with similar studies. Companies usually have to perform two or three large (so-called Phase III) studies in order to license a new drug. Very often these pivotal studies have virtually identical designs. If a journal has already published the results of one pivotal trial, it is unlikely to accept another. Since such trials often take place in different locations, a better strategy is to consider the journal's geographic reach and readership, for example submitting the North American study to a US journal, and the European one to a European journal.

■ House style

Virtually all journals (except a few electronic ones that do not invest in any copy editing) will impose their own (so-called 'house') style on your article before publication. House style includes spelling options (e.g. US versus UK, -ise versus -ize), conventions on abbreviations (e.g. how e.g. is punctuated), and typographic style for headings. There is no point in resisting this or trying to revert to your original version on the proofs. However, there is also no need to try to make your submission conform exactly to your target journal's style by using the same format for headings, etc. Although this might make you look keen and show that you have researched the journal thoroughly, most publishers actually prefer to receive simple text without fancy styles, as word processing codes usually have to be replaced with typesetting commands, so heavily formatted text may actually slow the process down. That is not to say that you should not follow the 'Instructions to authors', especially the preferred reference style (which will be simple if you have invested in bibliographic software), but, having done this, you need not try to make your typescript look exactly like a published paper.

House wine and house dressing are outside the scope of this book but may, if used judiciously, ease the publication process especially if they ensure that authors have time to get to know one another and discuss their publications in congenial surroundings. Many publication problems arise through lack of communication, so the more everybody can talk and get to know other team members, the smoother the process is likely to be.

I

■ ICMJE; *see* International Committee of Medical Journal Editors

■ Impact factors

Impact factors (IFs) are a measure of how often a journal's papers get cited. This is not a bad idea in itself, but, unfortunately, many academic institutions attach undue importance to IFs and use them to assess the importance of individual publications or researchers, which they were never designed to do. Some journal editors also get a bit over-excited about their IF. So, although it is tempting to say you should ignore them, you need to understand their misuse.

Journal IFs are published each year by the Institute of Scientific Information (ISI). The ISI is a commercial organisation (part of Thomson Reuters) which produces *Current Contents* and the *Science Citation* Index – it also charges publishers large amounts for each year's IF listings. For details *see* http://thomsonreuters.com

IFs are calculated by dividing the number of times a journal is cited in a given year by the number of full papers it has published in the previous two years. Letters and abstracts are not included in the denominator, although, of course, they may be cited – so journals that publish a lot of these may have inflated IFs. Journals are grouped into subjects (e.g. dermatology, general medicine) and ranked by IF. The prestigious general journals (e.g. *NEJM, The Lancet*) have much higher IFs than specialist journals.

While it is quite interesting to see how journals rank, there is probably only a very rough correlation between the whole journal's IF, and the impact of a single publication. It is possible that a few papers in the highest IF journals are never cited at all, while others become classics, so the average is a pretty crude statistic. Nevertheless, some universities rate the output of a department or researcher by multiplying the number of their publications by the IF of the journal in which they appeared. In some countries an individual needs a certain number of such publication 'points' before s/he can be appointed to the next grade (e.g. a professorship). This has the unfortunate effect of increasing the attractions of **guest authorship** (i.e. including colleagues' names on papers although they have contributed little or nothing to the research) and of making the IF the most important criterion for academics when selecting a journal.

Although the IF is one factor to bear in mind, it is a mistake to forget about the journal's readership, acceptance rate, time to publication, etc. when selecting a **target journal**. Great emphasis on IF can lead to academics insisting on submitting papers to journals that are unlikely to accept them, which often wastes time. It may also cause disagreements among authors if some want to hold out for the highest IF while others (or the study's sponsors) are more interested in the speed of publication or some other criterion.

The current IF listings are only available at a high price from ISI, who guards its copyright fiercely. However, some websites make previous years' rankings available (perhaps illegally) (e.g. http://www.bio21.bas.bg/ibf/IF99.txt or http://abhayjere.com/impactfactor.aspx).

You may also be able to discover a journal's current IF from its website or by making an enquiry to its editorial office.

Journal IFs vary between specialties, so if you are considering more than one target audience it is unwise to try to compare journals from different areas. (For example, if you wanted to publish a study on childhood asthma, you should consider the IFs of paediatrics journals separately from those for respiratory medicine – the rank order is a more reliable guide to a journal's influence than the numerical value of its IF – although, of course, if your sole aim is to choose the journal with the highest IF then there's no harm shopping around.)

Sadly, there is a correlation between IF and rejection rate – hence picking the journal with the highest IF will often increase your chance of rejection.

If co-authors cannot agree on a target journal, they might agree to the following compromise. The first choice journal will be one with a high IF (thus probably also a high rejection rate) but also a relatively rapid time to reject (e.g. one that rejects a large proportion of submissions after **in-house review**). If you get rejected, honour will have been satisfied, but you won't have wasted too much time. Everyone must agree (before submission to the first journal) that, if the paper is rejected by the first journal, it will be submitted (straightaway, and without further prolonged discussion) to a second journal with a greater chance of acceptance.

If all authors are determined to get the most IF points from a paper, you can work your way down the ranking until your paper is accepted. But, even the most assessment-conscious academic usually gets disheartened after a couple of rejections, and it gets harder to revise a paper the further you are from doing the research, so this strategy could, paradoxically, result in everybody getting fed up and the paper never being published (so no IF points for anybody). It is far better to agree your target audience, research your target journal carefully, be realistic about your chances of acceptance and regard the journal's IF as a side issue.

If you already know the IFs of all the journals in your specialty or can quote any impact factor to two decimal places, this is a strong indication that you are seriously over-stressed in your struggle for promotion or your department's research assessment exercise and need to take a holiday.

Getting clever with impact factors

Some editors get very competitive about their journal's IF and have even been known to try to inflate their figures by devious means. For example, a few editors have been caught demanding that authors include a certain number of citations to their own journal. While this is not considered good form among journal editors, authors should take note. Since journal editors like citations to their own journal, you might curry favour by including as many as possible. Don't overdo this, or include irrelevant references just because they come from the target journal, but it probably won't do any harm if you slip in a couple of citations of review articles or previous studies from the journal in your introduction. Apart from raising the journal's IF, including citations from previous publications is also a sign that you have selected your target journal with care, and may provide some reasons why the editor should publish your work, especially if it complements something the journal has already published.

Smith R (1997) Journal accused of manipulating impact factor. *BMJ*. **314**: 463.

EASE statement on inappropriate use of impact factors (2007) http://www.ease.org.uk/statements/index.shtml

■ IMRAD structure

Acronym for Introduction, Methods, Results and Discussion, used to describe the conventional structure of a scientific paper.

■ Indexing

Publishing in a journal that is indexed in the major databases will increase the chances of your paper being identified in literature searches. The most widely used database is **Medline**, produced by the US National Library of Medicine and available (free of charge) at http://www.ncbi.nlm.nih.gov/PubMed.

However, by no means all medical journals are included on Medline, and non-English language publications are particularly poorly represented. Other databases such as Embase (www.embase.com), Scopus (http://info.scopus.com) and BIOSIS (http://thomsonreuters.com/content/PDF/scientific/BIOSIS_Factsheet.pdf) include more titles, but charge a search fee so they tend to be available only at libraries and academic institutions, thus limiting access to serious and well-funded researchers. Choosing a journal that is included in Medline may therefore increase the accessibility of your publication.

Journals often ask for key words to help the indexing services classify articles correctly; it is therefore worth spending a few moments to select the best ones – *see* **key words** for more details.

■ Informal review

In your efforts to involve all the right **(key) people** and to jump through the hoops created by peer review it is easy to overlook informal review. Much of this book is about making sure a publication is reviewed by the right people at the right time, but you should also consider adding some extra, informal review steps. If parts of the submission are written by non-native English speakers, or even if they are written by several native speakers with different styles, it may be helpful to get a review from a native-speaking writer or editor. If you have access to information specialists or librarians they may be prepared to check your references. People outside your subject area such as husbands, wives or even cooperative children, can sometimes spot flaws in the logic or ways in which a paper could be made more accessible to a wider audience. Lay people are good at asking probing questions such as 'Why does this matter?' or 'Why did you do this?' which can help structure the introduction or discussion. *See also* Table 1.1, p. 4.

The secret of using informal review is to give very clear instructions. Explain to the potential reviewer exactly why you are asking them to read the paper and what you would like them to do, and give them a deadline. The timing of informal review is also important. There is no point doing a final check for grammar and spelling on sections that are likely to be rewritten. If you approach colleagues or investigators outside the writing group for their input you must also be clear about what rewards they can (and should not) expect – in particular, make it clear that their contribution will not lead to authorship if that is the case. If informal reviewers have been particularly helpful you should consider mentioning them in the **acknowledgements**.

For more information *see* the chapter on informal review in:

Wager E, Godlee F and Jefferson T (2002) *How to Survive Peer Review*. BMJ Books, London.

■ In-house review

Journals that employ several editors and receive many submissions often reject a considerable proportion of manuscripts after in-house review. This means that average times to rejection are shorter than those for acceptance. *See* **review process** and Chapter 3 'How long will it take?' (pp. 13–16) for more details.

The purpose of in-house review is to reduce the burden on external reviewers by sifting out submissions that are unsuitable for a particular journal. Editors rejecting papers during in-house review are most concerned about whether the findings are likely to interest their readers and whether the article fits the journal's scope rather than whether it follows reporting guidelines or the study was well executed. Editors (especially full-time ones) are generally not experts on your particular topic but do know what sort of articles they like to publish. If you are rejected after in-house review you therefore do not receive detailed criticism of your research or suggestions on how to improve your paper, but usually just a note saying 'sorry, it's not for us'. If you have failed to excite the editor sufficiently to warrant external review it probably means you have selected the wrong journal, so there is little point in appealing, and it is usually better to follow your **back-up plan** and submit to another journal. As the *BMJ* notes 'If the editors . . . have decided that your paper is not sufficiently interesting or important for *BMJ* readers, there may be no point in trying to appeal'. However, you might consider revising your paper to make sure you have explained why your research was interesting and important in the hope that you can convince another editor of its merits.

■ Initials; *see* names

■ Instructions to authors (contributors)

However helpful this book might be, there is no substitute for reading your target journal's instructions. Many journals now publish instructions on their websites, so you do not even need to leave the comfort of your office or lab. Read the instructions as soon as you select your target journal, then again before you prepare the submission package.

It is easy to get irritated by journal requirements, especially if you are already in a bad mood because your paper has been rejected by your first choice journal. If necessary, go and have a cup of coffee (or something stronger), or wait until you are feeling calmer, then tackle them like you would an exam question, making sure you have answered every point. If possible, get into a frame of mind that allows you to take pedantic pride in getting every little detail right. This will not guarantee acceptance but it should make a good impression on the editor and reviewers and certainly will not damage your chances.

■ Internal review

Virtually everybody has a boss or employer who will need to see papers or abstracts before submission so, unless all the authors are self-employed and self-funded, internal review is inevitable. In the case of big drug companies, this internal review may be complex and time-consuming. When you are planning a publication, try to find out what review steps will be needed and roughly how long they will take. Large companies usually have standard times (or targets) for review. It is also important to establish at what stage the various reviews should take place, and which can take place in parallel (to save time) rather than sequentially.

If you are collating comments you will also need to understand which changes take precedence. Some companies have a formal hierarchy for this, which, although it looks bureaucratic, is actually very helpful for an external writer or editor who then knows that, for example, changes suggested by the global legal department are sacrosanct, while comments from the Ruritanian marketing department can be ignored if they clash with others.

If you are designing a review process, it is best to aim for a pyramid structure, which involves lots of people at the early (e.g. outline stages), and gradually fewer and fewer people (apart, of course, from the authors) at the later stages.

If you are writing-up sponsored research, check your contract or investigators' agreement to see whether the sponsor wishes to review any planned submissions (they usually do), and, if so, how much time they need for this (60 days is not uncommon). Even if this is not stated in your contract, it is courteous to let the sponsor comment on any planned publications.

■ International Committee of Medical Journal Editors (ICMJE)

Also known as the Vancouver Group. An influential group of medical journal editors who first met in Vancouver in 1978 and who periodically issue guidance and pronouncements. The group has produced several editions of the 'Uniform Requirements for Manuscripts Submitted to Biomedical Journals' (the latest is available at www.icmje.org).

The initial impetus behind these requirements was the premise that authors should not have to format papers differently for different journals. (Remember that most papers were still produced on typewriters in the 1970s.) The theory is that, if you follow the requirements, your manuscript should be acceptable to any of the 500 or so journals that have signed up. However, editors now expect authors to be equipped with computers (not typewriters) so individual journal requirements and electronic submission systems are increasingly diverse and the optimistic view of achieving uniformity seems, paradoxically, to be increasingly unrealistic.

The original meeting place gave its name to the Vancouver style of references in which citations are numbered in the text and listed by their order of appearance in the reference list. However 'Vancouver style' is a generic term and there are endless subtle variations on this theme such as how many authors are listed before you use *et al.*, the punctuation of authors' names, and whether journal names are abbreviated.

Considering how easy it is to format references using bibliographic software there is really no excuse for not following the exact style of your target journal. Similarly, the 'Uniform Requirements . . .' do not tell you exactly how to structure an **abstract**, whether **key words** are used, etc. Although it should not matter, it does not do any harm to show that you have researched your target journal (and are not on the rebound from another) by formatting your submission precisely to the individual journal's style.

However, although the uniformity of the requirements may be a trap for the lazy, you should certainly read the ICMJE's more general statements about authorship, conflict of interest, etc. as they provide much useful information and insight into the way that editors feel about these things.

The current members of the ICMJE are the editors of:

- *Annals of Internal Medicine*
- *BMJ (British Medical Journal)*
- *CMAJ (Canadian Medical Association Journal)*
- *Croatian Medical Journal*
- *Journal of the American Medical Association*
- *Journal of the Danish Medical Association*
- *The Lancet*
- *Medical Journal of Australia*
- *Nederlands Tijdschrift voor Geneeskunde (Dutch Journal of Medicine)*
- *New England Journal of Medicine*
- *New Zealand Journal of Medicine*
- *Norwegian Medical Journal.*

but at their 2009 meeting, the ICMJE members agreed to invite applications to extend their rather exclusive membership by a couple more journals.

■ International Society for Medical Publication Professionals (ISMPP)

While medical writers organisations (such as **AMWA**) date back to the 1940s, publication planners didn't have their own society until 2005, when ISMPP (pronounced 'iz-map') was founded. Since then it has grown to include over 800 members and has well-attended meetings, in the US (until now), with plans for a European meeting in 2010. If you have a publications role in a drug or medical device company, or a specialist agency, you should consider joining so you can meet other people working in the area and keep abreast of new developments. ISMPP has also developed a credentialling system so you can even get letters after your name if you pass their exam. For more information *see* www.ismpp.org.

■ Investigators' agreements

This is an ideal place to set out the publication policy, including data ownership and authorship criteria. Starting to discuss the publication strategy in the early stages of the research process is also helpful, even if many details cannot be finalised until the data have been analysed. Thinking about the publication(s) before you start a study may also help to plan your research and ensure that you generate publishable results. *See* **contracts** and **publication agreements** for more details.

■ ISRCTN (International Standard Randomised Controlled Trial Number)

This trial register was originally set up by the company that published the **BioMed Central** journals but it was later transferred to a not-for-profit foundation. Although it meets the International Committee of Medical Journal Editors' requirements for an acceptable place to register clinical trials it does not include a results database and does not meet the requirements of **FDAAA** (the US law passed in 2007 which, effectively, required most trials to be registered on the US website **ClinicalTrials. gov**). Lacking government money (unlike ClinicalTrials.gov), ISRCTN has to charge a small administrative fee to registrants (although it is free to search), which is another reason why it may be doomed to obscurity. Which is a shame, because although ClinicalTrials.gov currently does an excellent job, the effective monopoly of a single register funded by one government (in this case the USA) is a bit scary and some people would prefer trial registration to be controlled by a more neutral, international organization.

J

■ Journal choice

This is the single most important decision within your publication strategy. Choice of journal will affect:

- what formats are available
- your chance of acceptance
- how long you have to wait for a decision
- the length of time from acceptance to publication
- who will read your work (at least initially)
- who will have access to your work via the web
- how your work is published (i.e. electronically, in print, or both)
- how your work is presented (e.g. how much copy editing is done at the journal)
- the visual appearance of your work (e.g. page layout, journal house style)
- how your research is perceived.

In a truly rational and scientific world, authors would sit down with a list of all available journals and information about all these variables and calculate the correct answer (and I would probably be out of a job because nobody would need my advice or want to read this book). However (and luckily for me), real life is messy, it is often hard to get all the information you need and, even faced with good evidence, human beings make subjective decisions. If you, your co-authors and other key players can agree on the choice of target journal (and, very importantly, also on the second choice) amicably over a few beers, then that is fine. But for a more logical (and alcohol-free) approach follow these steps.

1 Agree the **target audience** for your publication – this will usually include the readers' discipline, degree of specialisation and location, e.g. European family doctors with an interest in research, or North American cardiologists.
2 Scan the library, the internet and reference sections of related papers to develop a 'long-list' of possible journals likely to be read by your target audience.
3 Read the journals' instructions to authors to check whether these journals meet your needs in terms of the **formats** and any other restrictions such as article length. Eliminate any that do not.
4 Scan recent issues of possible journals to get an idea of the scope, coverage and **hot topics**. Do not rely on the journal **title** to determine this.
5 Decide how important the following factors are to you and the other **key players**, not forgetting the research sponsor:
   – speed of publication
   – journal reputation (e.g. **impact factor**)
   – publication medium (print or electronic)
   – accessibility (e.g. **indexing, Open Access journals**).

   Ideally, you should be able to agree on a ranking for all four factors – however, if different parties have different **expectations** (e.g. the sponsor wants to publish as quickly as possible but the first author wants to aim for the journal with the highest impact factor), then you should try to agree on the top two and seek a strategy that can satisfy both.
6 Gather as much information as you can on these criteria (or, at least on your top two). You will probably already know how the journal is published (print, web, etc.) and it is relatively easy to discover how accessible it is (e.g. whether it is **Open Access**, or is included in **Medline** or **PubMed Central**). It can be more difficult to discover how long journals take to reach decisions and to publish – *see* **decision times** and **lead time** for more details. Check recent issues in case the journal publishes submission and acceptance dates for articles – these are probably more reliable than targets mentioned in general information.
      Remember that the actual time to publication will depend not only on the speed of processing at your first target journal, but also on whether it accepts your paper. You therefore need to consider your chance of acceptance. *See* **acceptance rates** for more details.
      Reputation or prestige is, by definition, a subjective judgement, of which the **impact factor** is an imperfect measure. Asking colleagues or people who work in your field what they think of different journals is probably more useful. You should also gather incidental information that might affect your decision, such as having good contacts with the editor or members of the **editorial board**, knowing that the journal plans a theme issue that coincides with your interests, or seeing that the journal has recently published a related study.

7 At last, you will be in a position to draw up your short-list. You should have identified some journals that are likely to reach your target audience, accept the type of publication you have in mind and meet your other criteria to various extents. You should tabulate this information and share it with the key players who will have to make the decision. If you have succeeded in getting agreement on your priorities (step 5) it should be a relatively simple task to select the journal that best meets everybody's needs, with a runner-up as second choice. Lastly, if you are selecting journals for several projects (e.g. to create a product publication strategy), try to spread your choices over several journals and avoid submitting two similar studies (e.g. a North American and a European pivotal Phase III trial) to the same journal. If you have a budget but lack the time or inclination to research target journals you can purchase information from communication agencies or specialist companies offering publication planning tools such as **DataVision** and **PeerView**.

■ Journalists; *see* Media relations

K

■ Key message(s)

Every publication should have a message, or perhaps two. This message (or messages) should be discussed and agreed among the authors. If an external writer is brought in to develop a publication, the key message is one of the most important parts of the brief.

Defining your key message before you start to write will help to focus your writing and, in particular, know which details should be stressed, and which can be omitted. In this respect publications are different from the reports written for regulatory agencies, which must contain every detail of the research. Authors and writers need to exercise scientific and moral judgement in choosing what data to include in a publication. The distinction between a persuasive and focused paper and a biased or unrepresentative one is a fine one, and you should not let enthusiasm for your message slip over into 'spin'. However, it is a mistake to imagine that the perfect scientific paper is one without a message since such papers are likely to confuse and bore readers.

As a scientist or clinician you are entitled to hold opinions about what your findings mean, and expected to express them, especially in the discussion section. If you are preparing a publication jointly, or several authors are preparing different publications, it is very important that all contributors agree on the key messages so that their writing has some chance of hanging together to form a consistent whole, and so that different papers from the same project do not overlap.

Do not make the mistake of confusing the topic (or title) with the key message. For example, the topic of a study might be the safety of Wunderdrug in patients with diabetes. This tells you about the study but does not provide sufficient focus for writing it up. A message, like a sentence, needs a verb (i.e. a word indicating action). Thus, the message might be 'Wunderdrug does not cause hypoglycaemia in patients with diabetes' or 'Patients receiving Wunderdrug have normal liver function'.

Further judgement is needed in deciding how many publications should be derived from a single piece of research. For clear communication, and to keep within journal stipulations on length, each paper should have no more than two messages. If you and your co-authors believe there are three or more messages, you should consider splitting the publication, but be careful to avoid **redundant publication** and **salami science**. Some studies divide quite naturally into sections such as efficacy and **economic (health outcomes) evaluations**. Similarly, secondary (*post hoc*) analyses may be best presented as separate, secondary papers – but, in this case, make sure the main paper is referenced and try to make it clear to readers that both papers refer to the same study by including a clear **trial identifier**.

If you are preparing a plan for multiple publications the key messages for each publication should be clearly stated. If you are a professional writer being briefed about a study, remember that a key message needs a verb and be prepared to challenge vague statements such as 'this paper is about the efficacy of Wunderdrug'.

If there is no chance of all authors discussing a publication face-to-face, then circulating an **outline** can be a good way to generate discussion (and, with luck, agreement) on the key message(s).

■ Key people / players

The really important people in developing any publication are its authors. Make sure you have included everybody who qualifies (and read the section on **authorship** if you are in doubt). Remember, too, that other people such as your boss, or representatives from the funding organisation, may need to be involved. Allow sufficient time for everybody to comment on planned publications and try to work out the most efficient way of gathering comments and deciding who sees what, and when.

While all authors should have ample opportunity to contribute to a publication it may also help to identify 'key people' among the authors. Ideally, the entire writing group will meet to discuss the planned publication at various stages, for example developing the outline and agreeing the final version. However, it is sometimes impossible for everyone to meet face-to-face, and telephone conferences with more than five people can be frustrating and unproductive. In such cases, there may be a temptation to work more closely with one or two of the authors, and have slightly less contact with the others. This pattern is rarely a strategic decision, but sometimes arises because of difficulties of working across different time zones.

Working with an 'inner' and 'outer' writing group can cause problems and delays if the 'inner' group does not include everybody with strong views about the publication. If the 'inner' group takes decisions without consulting the others, this is unlikely to lead to good relations, and may even cause delays if the authors who were not consulted insist on major changes at a late stage. Try to avoid this situation by making sure everybody comments on the outline, so there are no surprises when a draft is produced.

■ Key words

Many journals ask authors to identify a few key words. These are designed to help the indexing services (such as **Medline**) classify papers correctly. Check the 'Instructions to authors' guidance notes for specific requirements but, in the absence of these, consider using the Medical Subject Headings (MeSH) used by Medline.

Unless you are very familiar with **MeSH headings** check before you select, as they can be idiosyncratic or old-fashioned. Bear in mind that most major Medline subject headings were selected in the mid-1960s and, in order to ensure consistent searchability, have not changed since then, although new terms have been added. Thus, you won't find 'proton pump inhibitors' as a recognised term, but these are categorised as 'anti-ulcer agents'.

The best way of checking MeSH headings is via the **PubMed** website (http://www.ncbi.nlm.nih.gov/PubMed).

L

■ Last author

See **order of authors** for a full discussion of this subject. In many disciplines the position of last author is endowed with special status and may be competed over almost as fiercely as the first. However, this status has never been defined, and probably varies between countries and specialties. Although the **International Committee of Medical Journal Editors' (ICMJE)** (Vancouver) criteria clearly state that obtaining funding or overall supervision of a department does not, alone, merit authorship, the last place has often been reserved for just such a person. *See* **guest authors** for more details. The trend for journals to list individuals' contributions rather than just their names and titles may reduce the prevalence of undeserving guest authors, but it is too early to tell whether it will abolish the jostling for last place.

In some cases, the **corresponding author** or **guarantor** occupies the last position but, again, there is no rule about this. While authors often appear to know what is so special about being last on the list, readers may, of course, be happily ignorant of this convention, or may apply the traditions of their own specialty, which may be different from those of the authors. The only rule is to discover all authors' understandings and expectations and to try to agree the order of authors amicably.

■ Late breaker abstracts

Submission deadlines are sometimes so long in advance of major conferences that there is a danger that only rather old research gets presented. Some meetings therefore allow 'late breaker abstracts' for new findings. You may have to provide evidence that your data were not available by the regular submission deadline, you are likely to be restricted to a **poster presentation**, rather than an **oral** one, and your **abstract** may not appear in the conference book, or may appear in a separate section, but it is worth enquiring if your target meeting permits late breakers if you have a genuine problem in hitting the submission deadline.

■ Lead time

(Pronounced like a dog leash, not like the heavy element.)

This is the time between acceptance and publication. It varies hugely from almost nothing (for electronic journals) to several months. Lead time may be an important factor in your choice of journal if it is important to have copies of your article by a certain date (e.g. for a big conference). However, since accepted articles may be cited as being 'in press', you may be more concerned about the **decision time**.

Some journals publish the acceptance date at the bottom of an article – in this case you can easily work out the average lead time. If this information is not available and you need to discover it, you should consult the website or contact the editorial office.

Many, but by no means all, journals publish accepted articles on their websites before they appear in print. Such articles are listed as 'epub ahead of print' on Medline. Electronic posting of the final version is considered to be publication and in some journals the electronic rather than the print version is now considered the definitive one. However, if you want **offprints** you will also need to know when the printed version will appear. Articles can be cited with a permanent (and useful) reference even before they have been assigned page numbers thanks to the **DOI system**.

Long delays between acceptance and publication were largely caused by editors accepting more articles than they had room to print. This caused queues which, in theory at least, should have been abolished by **electronic publication**. However, even now some journals still work to fixed page budgets and as recently as 2009 I got caught out by a journal with an eight-month lead time as I foolishly believed such dinosaurs were long extinct.

See Chapter 3 'How long will it take?' (pp. 13–16) for more details.

■ Legends; *see* figure legends

■ Letters to the editor

■ Writing

Journals publish two distinct types of letters: those that comment on published material, and those that contain new research findings. Some indexing systems treat these differently (usually including the latter but ignoring the former). You should therefore check the journal (and, if necessary the indexing system) before considering using a letter to present new findings. Research letters may be a useful format for studies with straightforward methods that can be compressed into a strict word limit. The acceptance rate and speed of publication for research letters are often slightly better than those for full articles.

The more traditional correspondence column can be useful to draw attention to your own publications or to offer supplementary information pertinent to the point being discussed. However, most journals accept letters only if they relate to something the journal has published. Some also set a time limit for receiving such letters (e.g. three weeks after the original publication in *NEJM*) which means you need to keep up to date with the literature, and be prepared to respond quickly.

■ Responding

If your publication stimulates letters that the journal plans to publish you will normally be given the opportunity to respond. If they receive several letters, print journals usually try to publish them together, along with the author's response. Production schedules mean that this correspondence often appears several months after the original publication (at least for print journals), but the journal may not give you much time to prepare a response, since letters are usually slotted into issues after other sections, so the decision to publish them is usually taken shortly before publication. This also means that you may not see a proof of your response, or may receive only a **galley** (not a **page**) **proof**.

In contrast, a few journals (notably the *BMJ* and *PLoS*) use their websites to encourage rapid, electronic responses. Authors may choose to respond to each letter individually or even enter into a dialogue with the responder. The corresponding author will usually be alerted when responses are posted – and it is a nice idea to let other authors know.

Try to address the points made by correspondents as succinctly and politely as possible (journal editors do not want letters that are long or defamatory) and consult your co-authors before you reply. It may help to treat the letters in the same way that you would approach reviewers' comments. In other words, take a deep breath, calm down, and try to be as objective as possible. Nobody likes having their interpretation called into question or flaws in their research brought to light, but remember that this is the way that science is meant to proceed, and at least the letter proves that somebody has read your paper and considers your work sufficiently interesting to comment on it.

M

■ Masked review; *see* blinded review

■ Meat extenders

A term coined by Ed Huth (former editor of *Annals of Internal Medicine*) to describe the act of 'blending data from one study with additional data to extract yet another paper that could not make its way on the second set of data alone'.[1] Thus, a form of **redundant publication**. But it raises the question of why this form of malpractice inspired such meaty metaphors (*see* **salami science**).

1 Huth E (1986) Irresponsible authorship and wasteful publication. *Ann Intern Med*. **104**: 257–9.

■ Media relations

A good publication strategy, especially one for a commercial product or major re-search project, should be accompanied by a broader communication strategy covering plans for working with the press (newspapers, television, radio, etc.). Except in the smallest of organisations, the nerdy scientific stuff (i.e. journal articles) and trendy media bits (i.e. public relations or PR) are usually handled by different people, with different hairstyles and pay packages but it makes sense if these two worlds communicate. In particular, publication planners need to make sure that the PR folk don't get over-enthusiastic and issue **press releases** before publication which might seriously mess up your chances of getting into a good journal. However, people involved with publications should share their plans so that the PR people can do their job and seize appropriate opportunities for corporate trumpet-blowing. Many of the major journals and publishers have their own press departments who are happy to cooperate over issuing press releases and editors are delighted when their publications get picked up by the general media.

Journalistic interest in presentations at meetings is less straightforward, especially if your results have been submitted to or accepted by, but not yet published in, a major journal. Check the journal's press embargo policies carefully and make sure you do not fall foul of them. Some journals even expect you to withdraw presenta-tions from conferences once they have accepted your paper – but others are more relaxed about this. Just occasionally, you may be able to orchestrate the perfect combination of a presentation at a big conference occurring simultaneously (or just hours before) publication in a prestigious journal with joint press activities. Such impressive choreography requires exciting results, a cooperative journal and a fair bit of luck with your timing.

Editors accept that journalists may attend scientific meetings and report the most interesting findings. However, they do not welcome authors (or their institutions or companies) actively seeking press coverage by holding **press conferences** or issuing press releases before a full paper is published. Since abstracts are considered to be in the public domain, it is acceptable to give these to journalists who request information but providing slides or copies of posters is risky as it could lead to extensive coverage that a journal would consider to be **prior publication**.

■ Medical writers

See Chapter 4.

If a professional writer works on a manuscript, their involvement, and more importantly who paid for it, should always be acknowledged. Most journals follow the **International Committee of Medical Journal Editors' (ICMJE)** criteria for authorship and do not consider a writer who has not been involved in the design or conduct of the study as an author. However, one or two journals interpret the criteria differently and feel that anybody who helps write a manuscript must be an author (*see* **Acknowledgements** for details). Professional writers whose contribution is properly acknowledged (either in the acknowledgements, as contributors or even as authors) are not **ghost writers** (because they are visible). However, this rather insulting term is often used and sometimes gets confused with **ghost authors,** which constitute a quite different spooky problem.

■ Medline

A bibliographic database, run by the US National Library of Medicine, covering around 5000 medical journals with entries from 1949. Medline is probably the most widely used, although not the most comprehensive, database for doctors searching the literature since it is available free on the internet via **PubMed** (http://www. ncbi.nlm.nih.gov/PubMed). For this reason, articles in journals that are included in Medline are more likely to be retrieved (or at least their abstracts read) by researchers than those that are not listed, so inclusion in Medline is an important consideration when choosing a **target journal.**

Medline includes the title and author details and usually an abstract, but never the full text of an article. However, full text of some articles is now available on **PubMed Central** which can be searched from the same website.

■ Meeting choice; *see* congress / conference choice

■ Meetings (of the writing group)

The fastest, most efficient and probably most pleasant way to discuss and get agreement on publication strategy is for the **writing group** to meet. If your budget and diaries permit, try to organise at least two meetings. The first should be held as soon as results are available. The purpose of this meeting is to agree the **key message(s)**, confirm the membership of the writing group and their tasks, and thus finalise the authors for each publication. Ideally, you should already have some idea of how many abstracts or papers you plan to publish and who they are aimed at. Now that you know the results you can firm up these plans and select your target and second-choice journals and target meetings. The decisions taken at this meeting will form the core of your publication strategy. Appoint somebody to take and circulate notes of decisions made and action points. Once the strategy is agreed, you should produce a detailed plan showing target dates for milestones such as first draft, review, submission, etc. *See* Chapter 3 'How long will it take?' (pp. 13–16) and Chapter 2 'Developing a publication plan for a multicentre study' (pp. 7–12) for more details.

The second meeting should take place when you have a reasonably mature draft and all **key players** have had a chance to contribute. The object of this meeting is to agree a final version for submission. Setting a date for the second meeting is harder than for the first, since there is little point in meeting if your paper still requires a lot of detailed work but you risk delaying submission if you wait too long. You should therefore schedule two or three possible dates at the first meeting and try to persuade members to keep them free.

If members of the writing group and all other key players can agree on the final wording of the submission by e-mail, you may not need a second meeting. However, if there are differences of opinion, a meeting is usually the swiftest way to resolve them. If a meeting is impossible, a telephone (or video) conference is the next best thing, and definitely preferable to infinite rounds of e-mail. Once again, appoint somebody to record decisions and circulate notes to all attendees and to any key players who could not take part.

■ MeSH headings

A system of Medical Subject Headings used to categorise entries by the US National Library of Medicine's **Medline** and used by some journals for key words. The best way to find MeSH headings is via the **PubMed** website: http://www.ncbi.nlm.nih.gov/PubMed which gives a complete list. Even if a journal does not specify that you should use MeSH headings for key words they are a good starting point and may help ensure your publication is correctly coded if it is listed on Medline.

■ Metrics

Cynics, according to George Bernard Shaw are people who know 'the price of everything and the value of nothing'. Sadly, this description applies to many bosses who don't understand the importance of publications. Even if you are lucky enough to work for a more enlightened manager, you are likely to have to justify your budget or your fees at some point, so you may need to resort to metrics (which is just a fancy term for measuring what you do).

However, unlike many other industrial processes, where it is relatively easy to demonstrate efficiencies and to prove the value of what you do, it is remarkably tricky to devise sensible metrics for publication activities. For example, if you measured the success of a team by how often they got papers accepted in their first target journal, this would probably ensure that they never submitted anything to the top journals with the lowest acceptance rates but the highest impact factors. Conversely, if you rate publications only by the impact factor of the journal in which they are published, this could encourage time-wasting strategies with unrealistic target journals.

Another problem in publication metrics is that it often makes good sense to hold back some publications while speeding up others. For instance, you should not publish secondary papers before primary ones, so setting fixed targets for all papers (e.g. aiming to submit all papers within four months of results becoming available) doesn't make sense. It also seems unfair to hold authors, writers or planners entirely responsible for delays caused by journals' peer review or production processes – although perhaps they should take some responsibility for choosing a slow journal in the first place.

Discussing metrics with people from other companies, for example at **ISMPP** or **The International Publication Planning Association (TIPPA)** meetings, may offer helpful insights, but don't expect companies to share all their performance secrets willingly. If your company takes part in 'benchmarking' (i.e. sharing data with a group of companies, usually via a consultant, to establish industry norms and identify best practice), you might be able to get information about how long companies take to publish their clinical trials, on average.

If you are an in-house publication team and need to justify your budget you can ask a couple of friendly agencies about their standard fees for producing various types of publication and use this to demonstrate your productivity. But trying to show that your publications are better than others, or that your publication strategy is top notch is always going to involve some subjective judgements, so don't expect this to be an easy or uncontroversial process. If you get into unproductive arguments, try using the George Bernard Shaw quote at the beginning of this section.

N

■ Names

Think about how the authors' names will appear in the journal, in references, and in indexes such as **Medline**. If you use the format 'full given name, surname' (e.g. John

Smith) this will appear as Smith, J in indexes and there will be no information about middle names. If you use the format 'initials, surname' (i.e. J E Smith) or 'first name, initials, surname' (i.e. John E Smith), the name will appear as Smith, J E in indexes and reference lists. It is up to the author to indicate how his or her name should appear, but most people prefer to use their full names, especially if short versions start with a different letter (e.g. my friends call me Liz, but I use Elizabeth for publications).

Take particular care with multi-part names or those in which the family name appears before the individual name. Most English language journals are not particularly good at handling Spanish or Chinese names.

Accents on names often disappear when you submit abstracts or papers electronically. There is not much you can do about abstracts, as you rarely see proofs, although you could try e-mailing the conference organisers; but for papers, check proofs carefully.

Indexing systems sometimes garble, or ignore, group names.[1] This is a shame, as it may discourage their use. To increase the chances of your paper being retrieved correctly, it is safest to include individual members of the **writing group** as well as a group name (e.g. M Barassment & N Continent on behalf of the DRIBBLE study group). Journals that list people's contributions and include a study **guarantor** always require individuals to be listed as well as a study group.

See also **order of authors, group authorship**

1 Dickersin K, Scherer R, Suci ES *et al.* (2002) Problems with indexing and citation of articles with group authorship. *JAMA.* **287**: 2772–4.

■ Nitpickers

Every place of work has somebody who can spot a typo at a hundred paces and delights in a misplaced apostrophe. If you handle them carefully, you can use such nitpickers to your advantage. The following rules will help:

- never show your first draft to a nitpicker
- if possible, wait until several other people have reviewed a manuscript before you ask a nitpicker to read it
- as with other reviewers, give the nitpicker clear information about the status of the manuscript, which parts cannot be changed, exactly what you would like him/ her to do, and by when.

Used this way, a keen-eyed reviewer, or somebody with a good sense of grammar and style can be an ally. Nitpickers should not be confused with **vicious reviewers** who make personal attacks and take pleasure in tearing apart other researchers' work. Although nitpickers can be annoying, remember that a really thorough **internal review** is usually less painful than a dressing down from the journal's reviewers and it may increase your chances of acceptance. Even though good science should shine through a poorly prepared manuscript, appearances do matter, and a polished paper is likely to impress reviewers and editors. *See* **proofs (page proofs)** – when nitpickers can be really useful.

■ Number of authors

The number of authors on each publication should be determined by established criteria. *See* **authorship** for more details. Whatever criteria are used, they must be applied equally to everybody involved with the study. Some sponsor companies, aware that readers' and reviewers' perceptions might be affected by seeing several employees on the author list, try to play down their involvement and may try to restrict the number of employee authors (or even forbid them altogether) creating **ghost authors**. It is up to the other authors to explain that this is unacceptable. The move from a simple **by-line** to the **contributorship** system may discourage this practice, since it may be apparent that a **key person** (e.g. a statistician) has been omitted.

The **International Committee of Medical Journal Editors' (ICMJE)** guidelines state that contributors who do not meet the authorship criteria should not be listed, and that all those who do meet the criteria should be included. **Good Publication Practice (GPP)** also encourages companies to apply criteria consistently to employees and external investigators (*see* p. 156).

Since all authors must contribute to the publication, in addition to their contribution to the research itself, establishing a **writing group** can help to distinguish those who qualify for authorship from other investigators.

Large studies may have many authors. However, as a general rule, the more authors there are, the longer a publication will take to develop. For short reports or case studies an interminable list of authors may stretch the credibility of readers and reviewers and raise suspicions of **guest authorship**.

Although it is rarely spelled out, the same authorship conventions apply for abstracts as for full papers. However, local investigators may sometimes be added to the author list if they are presenting findings at a local meeting.

■ Number of publications

Deciding how many publications you can squeeze out of your research is one of the most important strategic decisions you will have to make. Sadly, there is no simple formula to guide you. The findings of some enormous and important studies can be neatly summed up in a single paper, while other studies may warrant all sorts of secondary publications. For academics seeking to enrich their CVs, or companies hoping to promote their product, it may be tempting to try to produce masses of publications but if you overstep the limits of reasonableness you may stand accused of **salami science** or **redundant publication**. However tempting it may be to dream of dozens of publications, try to keep readers and editors in mind and think about what they want. It can be frustrating to have to piece together several bits of jigsaw that should really have been published as a whole. Also, if your strategy produces many overlapping papers, you may find that editors do not want to publish them, so you would have been better off with more modest ambitions.

O

■ Offprints

These are individual copies of a paper ordered before publication (as opposed to **reprints** which, strictly speaking, are printed separately, after the original version has been published; however, the terms are sometimes used interchangeably). Because they are printed at the same time as the complete journal, offprints are usually cheaper than reprints ordered after publication. Offprint order forms are usually sent with the proofs and must be returned quickly. You should therefore establish how many offprints are needed (by consulting all authors, the sponsor, and anybody else likely to want copies) as soon as the paper is accepted. Do not wait until the proofs arrive – large companies often take several weeks to sort out purchase orders or check how many copies their affiliate companies want and this could delay the proofs and therefore publication. Since the price of offprints usually depends on the length of the article you may not get an exact figure until page proofs are produced. However, you can get a price chart from the publisher and ask the editor in charge of production for an estimate of how many pages your article will fill.

Open Access journals may permit or even encourage you to print your own copies or to send electronic offprints (e.g. PDF files) but check with the journal before assuming that this is allowed.

■ Ombudsman / ombudsperson

One or two journals have appointed ombudsmen to hear grievances from disgruntled authors or readers. These ombudsmen are usually respected academics who are independent from the journal. Their role is to adjudicate in disagreements that cannot be settled satisfactorily by the editorial team. *See* **appeals** for more details.

Carter R (2004) Ombudsperson's eighth report. *The Lancet*. **364**: 402

Horton R (1998) The journal ombudsperson: a step toward scientific press oversight. *JAMA*. **280**: 298–9.

Both references describe *The Lancet*'s system.

■ Open Access journals

Journals can be categorised according to who pays for access to their contents. In the traditional funding model, journals make their full contents available only to those who have paid a subscription to the print or electronic versions, or those who pay for access to a particular item (sometimes called 'pay-per-view'). In contrast, Open

Access journals are freely available, on the web, to all readers, and authors usually pay a publication fee or **page charge**.

According to the Berlin declaration[1], Open Access journals must allow authors to retain copyright on their work and must deposit their contents in a permanent repository (e.g. **PubMed Central**) to ensure it doesn't disappear. Journals that meet these requirements usually refer to themselves as Open Access (with capital O and A) to distinguish themselves from other publications that may be freely available on the web but don't meet the other Berlin criteria.

The trend towards Open Access gathered momentum in the late 1990s with the expansion of electronic publishing. Open Access has some influential supporters especially among academic institutions who find it increasingly hard to pay journal subscription rates. Some large research sponsors (notably the US National Institutes of Health, Wellcome Trust and UK Medical Research Council) now require their studies to be published in Open Access journals. As a result, some commercial publishers have agreed to a compromise position of making all or part of their publications available some time after the initial publication. For example, you can access research papers (but not reviews or commentaries) from the *New England Journal of Medicine* on the journal website six months after they appear in the paper journal. Other publishers have responded by offering Open Access as an option to authors for a fee (usually between $1000 and $3000 per article, *see* for example, http://www.oxfordjournals.org/oxfordopen/)

When selecting a journal you should consider how accessible it is, especially if you want your work to be read beyond academic institutions or in resource-poor countries. Journals that have adopted the Open Access model include those from **BioMed Central** and the **Public Library of Science (PLoS)**.

1 Berlin Declaration (2003) http://www.oa.mpg.de/openaccess-berlin/berlindeclaration.html

Tamber PS, Godlee F and Newmark P (2003) Open access to peer-reviewed research: making it happen. *The Lancet.* **362**: 1575–7.

■ Open peer review

A review in which the reviewer's identity is revealed to the author(s). *See* **blinded (masked) review** and **review process** for details of other systems.

■ Oral presentations

Talks given at conferences are called oral presentations (following the curious scientific tradition of preferring long words to short ones). Since time is more limited than space most meetings accept relatively few submissions for oral presentations and the bulk are presented as posters. Talks are therefore considered more prestigious than posters and are more likely to generate media attention. However, some conferences allow authors to indicate their preference for an oral or poster presentation. Consider opting for a poster if the person who will present the research does not speak English fluently: remember that, as well as delivering the talk, the presenter will have to answer questions, and cannot always follow a script.

Good preparation is the key to a good talk and also permits co-authors to comment. Treat the slides like any other publication and make sure you get input from all **key players**. The presentation should be a team effort not an opportunity for the presenter to air his or her personal theories or pet interests. *See* **slides** for more details.

To avoid jeopardising the full publication, you should not distribute copies of your slides to journalists, although you may provide your abstract and answer their questions. Perhaps surprisingly, most journals do not consider a 'webcast' from a meeting to constitute prior publication.[1]

The key to obtaining an oral presentation is to craft a persuasive **abstract** but it is not always easy to convey your findings in a few words. Having a clear message and identifying the interests and needs of your audience are important factors for success. Having interesting results also helps.

1 Kassirer JP (1999) Posting presentations at medical meetings on the internet. *NEJM*. **340**: 803.

■ Order of authors

This can cause all sorts of problems and neither individual journals nor the **International Committee of Medical Journal Editors (ICMJE)** gives any advice on the subject. The main problem is that everybody thinks they know what the listing order implies but, in fact, conventions vary between disciplines and between countries.

Perhaps the only firm fact is that most people regard the first named author as the most important. The author/date (Harvard) reference system emphasises this by identifying publications by their first author in the text (e.g. Wager *et al.*, 2003).

The last position on the **by-line** sometimes indicates seniority or overall supervision. However, this is not universally true. *See* **number of authors** and **guest authors** if you are tempted to add a prestigious 'guest' to your author list.

Various systems have been devised for more democratic or transparent listing but, since you normally cannot explain what system you have used, readers are usually none the wiser. Listing by alphabetical order may seem fair if your name is Aaronson, but will probably be less attractive to Dr Zblinski (or even Ms Wager).

Some researchers have proposed mathematical formulae to determine author order.[1] However, these have not been widely adopted and are unlikely to solve your problems, since they rely on subjective assessments about who did what, and what each contribution is worth – which is usually what authorship disagreements are about.

The most practical advice is to discuss the order of authors as soon as you have agreed who will be listed. Discover the expectations and perceptions of all co-authors/contributors and try to reach an amicable agreement. Do not leave this to the final draft or just before the deadline for submission.

If a study will generate several publications you may be able to placate disgruntled co-authors by using different orders for each paper.

1 Hunt R (1991) Trying an authorship index. *Nature*. **352**: 187.

Bhopal RS, Rankin JM, McColl E *et al*. (1997) The vexed question of authorship: views of researchers in a British medical faculty. *BMJ*. **314**: 1009–12.

Bhopal RS, Rankin JM, McColl E *et al*. (1997) Authorship. Team approach to assigning authorship order is recommended. *BMJ*. **314**: 1046.

■ Organisations

Some journals retain close links with their parent organisation (usually an academic society). This may mean that they give priority to material presented at the society's meetings or from its members. Check these links when choosing your **target journal** to see if they could work for or against you.

Some meetings restrict abstract submission to members of the organising society, or require that a member sponsors every abstract. Check these requirements well before the submission deadline to prevent delays.

■ Outlines

Although you may be keen to rush into the first draft, preparing an outline of a planned publication is time well spent. The main advantage of an outline is that it allows you to decide on the contents of the paper and to get agreement from all **key players** before you commit time and effort to preparing a full draft. It is far better to discover differences in interpretation at this stage than after you have spent days writing a draft. The outline also bridges the gap between agreeing the **key messages**, which are, by definition, simplified and concise, and elaborating on these. An outline can also prevent overlaps or omissions and improve consistency when several people are writing a paper.

Even if you have circulated notes about the publication strategy, it is a good idea to re-state the main decisions (e.g. target audience, target journal and second choice journal) on the outline. You should also indicate important target journal requirements such as word limits and special formatting instructions, e.g. Abstract (structured, maximum 250 words).

All key players should review the outline, not just the authors. For some reason, people often pay less attention to reviewing an outline than to reviewing a full draft. You may therefore need to explain why you are circulating an outline and to remind key players that publication may be delayed if they raise major queries about the structure of the paper or the **key message(s)** after this stage.

■ Overlapping publications; *see* redundant publications

■ Ownership of data

This can be a thorny issue and it is therefore important that ownership is clearly set out in the **investigators' agreement** or **publication agreement**. Ownership of data should not be confused with **access to data**. Many research sponsors assert that data from a trial that they have funded belongs to them; even if this is the case, there should be a clause in the agreement that investigators will have access to the data and will be free to publish. The term 'data' can also have varying interpretations. It is a condition of most research that individual (unanonymised) patient data remain confidential and are not released to investigators. The only exceptions are accounts of serious adverse events which may, of necessity, contain information by which a patient could be identified. In practice, access to data usually therefore means access to the analysed (not raw) data set.

   Problems can arise if investigators want to perform additional (i.e. secondary) analyses. Ideally, all statistical analyses are agreed beforehand and set out in the **data analysis plan**. The sponsor and investigators should therefore discuss this and agree what analyses will (and will not) be done. If the results reveal unexpected findings it may be acceptable to do some secondary, explorative analyses. However, investigators must realise that sponsors usually do not have unlimited time or budgets for these. It is also important to get statistical advice about whether such analyses are meaningful.

P

■ Page budget

Most printed journals run to a page budget; in other words, the editor knows that each issue or volume of the journal must not exceed a certain length agreed with the publisher. This makes economic sense if printing and distribution are a major cost (which they are for traditional printed journals) and if the journal's income is largely derived from subscriptions that are paid in advance each year (so there is no way to go back for more money once it has been spent). However, page budgets can cause a lengthy **lead time** if editors accept more papers than they can publish each year. **Electronic publishing** has changed all this. Purely electronic journals have no limit on space and therefore no need for a queue of papers. Even journals that retain a print version may alleviate the problem of long lead times by making accepted papers available on their website before they appear in print.

■ Page charges

A **pay journal** usually charges authors around $1000 to $3000 per article for electronic publications. In the past, such journals, despite being peer reviewed, were criticised by editors of journals funded by subscriptions and advertising as a form of vanity publishing catering for the pharmaceutical industry. However, more recently, the scientific publishing community has been discussing the rights and wrongs of how journals are funded and the effects that different funding models have on the availability of research findings. There is now a move towards **Open Access journals** making papers available at no charge to readers via a website. However, even a wholly electronic journal incurs running costs and needs to employ staff to identify reviewers, administer the review process, etc. Instead of charging readers a subscription, Open Access journals charge authors or research sponsors. Some of these electronic Open Access journals attract high quality papers from both academic scientists and industry, and may have rejection rates and **impact factors** similar to those for traditional journals. The distinction between low quality pay journals and more respected journals is therefore blurring.

Since publication charges can be high, and tend to rise each year, check target journals' websites to ensure you have the latest details.

■ Pay journals

A journal funded by a publication fee (**page charge**) or reprints. These journals are also called 'controlled circulation journals' since they usually have no, or few, paid subscribers but are sent, instead, to a list of libraries and institutions chosen (i.e. controlled) by the publisher. The term is also applied to newspapers that are distributed freely to individual doctors and are funded by advertising. In common parlance, such newspapers are more often referred to as **freebies**, or less flatteringly, as 'throwaways'.

Pay journals are extremely useful if speed of publication is important, but as the name implies, you will have to pay for the service. Most offer review within one to three weeks, and, despite their high acceptance rates (of around 70–80%), this review can be surprisingly thorough. You can expect comments from two or three reviewers who, while they may not be big names in your field, will certainly know enough to spot flaws in your paper. As well as a rapid decision, most pay journals offer prompt publication. Electronic publication may be almost instantaneous after acceptance, with paper copies available shortly afterwards.

Pay journals have two systems for making money – they either charge a fee per printed page, or they insist that you buy a minimum number of reprints. In either case, you only pay if your paper is accepted.

Although pay journals do not have large numbers of subscribers, articles can reach your **target audience** by the distribution of reprints, via the journal website, or via bibliographic indexes such as **Medline**. Journals that are listed on Medline offer a distinct advantage to those that are not, since this provides a permanent record of your work and a means of other researchers contacting you even if they cannot get hold of the original journal.

Examples of pay journals are: *Clinical Therapeutics, Current Medical Research & Opinion, Acta Therapeutica* and *Clinical Drug Investigation*.

In the last few years, many purely electronic journals operating an 'author pays' model of Open Access have been established, e.g. by **BioMed Central** and the **Public Library of Science** (PLoS). These journals levy charges (currently $1000 to $3000 per paper) but also offer institutional subscriptions that allow researchers at participating institutions to publish without charge and waive charges for authors who cannot pay.

■ Peers

It has been claimed, probably by somebody who just received a damning rejection, that the truly original have no peers, but, for the rest of us, submissions are judged by reviewers whom journal editors consider our equals, or at least up to the job. Several authors have been unable to resist puns about peering into peer review, although, so far as I know, none have drawn analogies to the ermine-clad members of the UK House of Lords (and I am still unsure why they are called peers since they would seem to be definitely more equal than others).

A few journals ask authors to suggest people who might review their paper. This is a requirement for electronic submission to the **BioMed Central** journals, so you should think of some names before you submit. You should not propose anybody who has been involved with the research being reported, nor anybody at the same institution as the author(s). Some journals will follow authors' suggestions in most cases, while others chiefly use such information to enlarge their reviewer database. Unless your target journal practises **open peer review** you will probably never know if your suggestions have been followed.

Even when editors use a reviewer suggested by the author, they will almost certainly also approach at least one other reviewer from the journal's database. Although authors expect to be judged by their peers (i.e. people of similar standing), it has been known for senior researchers to delegate the job of reviewing to their juniors and they do not always inform the journal about this. While journal editors and authors might feel aggrieved about this (if they were aware of it), there is evidence[1] that younger scientists actually produce more conscientious and helpful reviews than older ones, so such delegation may not be entirely a bad thing.

If you feel that a reviewer has misunderstood your research, it might be worth writing an **appeal** to the editor, especially if another reviewer has recognised the merits of your paper. However, be careful to be as objective as possible, and avoid attacking the reviewer's education or intelligence (whether you know their identity or not). If the review was anonymous do not suggest that you know the reviewer's identity. For one thing, it undermines the principles of anonymous review and may make the editor uneasy, and for another, you might be wrong.

1 Black N, van Rooyen S, Godlee F *et al.* (1998) What makes a good reviewer and a good review for a general medical journal? *JAMA.* **280**: 231–3.

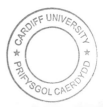

■ PeerView

A commercial company that provides detailed and comprehensive information about journals and conferences to assist companies in publication planning and also specialised publication planning software. *See* www.epeerview.com

■ Permissions

You need the copyright holder's permission to reproduce a figure, table or substantial chunk of text in a publication. Copyright law is rather vague about what constitutes a substantial amount of text but the UK Society of Authors advises that quotations of fewer than 400 words do not require permission. Remember that the author is not necessarily the copyright holder, so even if you wrote the original publication you may still need to get permission from the publisher. Ownership of copyright depends on the source. As a general rule, for subscription-based journals and for books, it tends to be the publisher. But **Open Access journals** usually have different arrangements under which the authors retain copyright.

Allow plenty of time to sort out permissions. Some publishers respond rapidly (Elsevier takes ten days), but some can take weeks or even months (e.g. the *Journal of Clinical Oncology* takes up to 30 working days). You will also need to think about your budget. Some publishers demand payment (often about $100 per figure) but fees vary depending on the planned use and could be substantially higher for commercial material or for electronic distribution.

You can usually find details about obtaining permission on the journal or publisher's website. In other cases, send your request to the publisher (not to the academic editor).

Although you should apply for permission as soon as possible, you cannot do this before you have selected your **target journal**, or have a rough idea of when the paper might be published, since most publishers request this information. You will also need precise details of what you hope to reproduce (e.g. the figure or table and page number, plus the full reference). Check that the item has not been taken from another publication (e.g. read the legend for any acknowledgements) and, if it has, track down the primary source and approach the original copyright holder, since the intermediate owner (i.e. the second journal or book publisher) is unlikely to be able to grant you permission.

Keep a copy of permission letters since some journals require these before they will publish your paper. You should also note any requirements for the way in which the permission is acknowledged.

■ Personal communications

If you want to quote something that somebody has said but not formally published you will probably need to resort to a 'personal communication'. First, check the instructions of your target journal to see if this kind of attribution is acceptable (some journals do not allow them).

Unlike reference citations, which usually give only the author's family name (e.g. Smith, 1999), personal communications usually indicate the first name (presumably to avoid misattribution to other people with the same surname). For example 'Up to 60% of people who attend publishing workshops fall asleep after lunch (personal communication: Liz Wager)'.

Some journals require even fuller details, for example *Circulation* demands details of the originating person's qualifications, *Blood* requires the person's affiliation and the method of communication (oral, written etc.). Some journals (e.g. *Journal of Antimicrobial Chemotherapy*) require a signature from anybody who is mentioned in this way. In any case, it is courteous to check with the person you wish to name, and they might even be able to provide a 'proper' reference if they have subsequently published their observation. If your target journal requires written evidence, or details such as the qualifications and affiliation of the quoted person, obtain these in good time so that they do not delay submission.

■ Pharmaceutical Research and Manufacturers of America (PhRMA)

If you are working for or with a US drug company you should be aware of the PhRMA Principles on Conduct of Clinical Trials and Communication of Clinical Trial Results which were issued in 2002 and revised in 2004 and 2009.

http://www.phrma.org/clinical_trials/

■ Placeholder abstracts

Some meetings accept abstracts that describe the design of a study but not the results. This can be tempting if the submission deadline is long before the meeting and you are confident of having exciting data to present. However, there are several dangers in submitting a placeholder. The first is that many meetings will simply reject such abstracts, so you will have wasted your time. The second is that, despite careful planning, you may not actually have results in time for the meeting. The third is that your results spring surprises so that **key players** cannot agree on their meaning in time for the meeting. Less scrupulous companies have sometimes withdrawn abstracts if results proved unfavourable, but this practice is unacceptable, since it constitutes **selective publication** and contributes to **publication bias**.

A better strategy is to submit to meetings with more convenient deadlines, or those that accept **late breaker abstracts**.

■ Plagiarism

In science one may progress, like Sir Isaac Newton, by 'standing on the shoulders of giants' but you should not conceal the acrobatics. In other words, it is acceptable (in fact, essential) to reference other works, but you must always acknowledge them and you should never copy sections from other publications and pass them off as your own work.

The Committee on Publication Ethics states 'all sources should be disclosed, and if large amounts of other people's written or illustrative material is to be used, permission must be sought'. *See* **permissions** for more details.

Remember that, in many cases, the author does not hold the **copyright** to work published in a journal or book. In such cases, strictly speaking, you will need permission to reproduce substantial sections of your own work. In practice, this certainly means obtaining permission to reproduce figures or tables.

Leaving aside the ethical and legal arguments, plagiarism (even self-plagiarism) is a sign of lazy writing. Every publication should have a unique **key message** and bolting together bits of other papers is not the most effective way of getting this across. If you need to describe a standard method it is usually better (and shorter) to reference the original work. If you are tempted to copy parts of other papers because you are not writing in your native language, you will produce a better paper if you write down your own ideas, however ungrammatical, and then ask a native speaker to edit them.

If you believe somebody has plagiarised your work you should alert your publisher before considering contacting the author or the publisher of the stolen version. One advantage of publishers holding the copyright of your work is that they are usually prepared to defend your case and advise you how to proceed.

A useful review can be found in:

Eaton L (2004) Plagiarism: the thin grey line. *BMJ Career Focus* 28. August. **329:** 85–6.

http://careerfocus.bmjjournals.com/cgi/content/full/329/7464/85

■ Planning

See Chapter 2 'Developing a publication plan for a multicentre study' (pp. 7–12) and Chapter 3 'How long will it take?' (pp. 13–16) for more details of this essential aspect of getting research published.

Remember that you need an agreed strategy before you can start to plan. Also, that the more detailed the plan (in terms of publication milestones and who is responsible for doing what) the more likely it is to be realistic and helpful. If you are working to tight deadlines (e.g. to get an abstract submitted) you should circulate the plan to all key players to make sure they can meet the timelines (e.g. they are not planning a holiday around crucial dates). If timelines change, keep everybody informed. If you are trying to coordinate multiple publications (e.g. a product publication strategy) then you might consider appointing a project manager whose sole responsibility is keeping the projects on track. In other cases, the lead author or professional writer can perform this role; but remember that being a brilliant scientist or communicator does not automatically make somebody a wonderful project manager.

■ PLoS; *see* Public Library of Science

■ Poster presentations

Abstracts submitted to conferences may be accepted for poster presentations. If the conference allows you to state a preference for oral or poster presentation this should form part of your publication strategy. Posters are generally considered less prestigious than an oral presentation but may be better if you lack confidence in spoken English. Another advantage of presenting work as a poster is that you can distribute copies of the poster at the meeting and send them to people who need to know the results. (Copies of posters are usually more informative than copies of slide sets.) However, you should avoid distributing copies of posters to journalists or widely to people who did not attend the conference, since extensive reporting of research could jeopardise full publication in a journal.

Preparing a successful poster is an art. Many companies and large institutions have design departments who can do this, or, if you have a budget, you can hire a graphic designer. While professionally prepared posters look attractive, they should not resemble promotional material. A discreet logo is acceptable, and maybe even using colours associated with a product, institution or company, but posters should be regarded as scientific communications and therefore should not make excessive use of brand names or other promotional devices. Reserve your creative talents for deciding how to present your data so that your **key messages** are rapidly and clearly communicated. Remember that most conference participants spend only a couple of minutes scanning each poster. Logical organisation, clear graphics and good use of colour can help get your message across.

Like slide sets and anything submitted to journals, ensure plenty of time for everybody to comment on the poster layout and content, and then allow sufficient time for poster production. Getting agreement on the draft contents before a professional designer starts work will help to keep your design costs within budget and avoid expensive and time-consuming amendments.

Conferences usually provide information about the size and orientation of posters. If you are working to a strict budget, get agreement on the number of handouts, whether these are colour or black and white, and check on different production methods (e.g. one large sheet, or separate sections, laminated or not) that will affect production costs. If you have to take a poster to a distant meeting think about airline baggage restrictions. If you do not want to risk consigning the poster to the hold (where it could get lost or damaged) you will need a format that can be carried as hand baggage.

Fraser J, Fuller L, Hutber G (2009) *Creating Effective Conference Abstracts and Posters in Biomedicine.* Radcliffe Publishing, Oxford.

■ Post-publication review and comments

Back in the good old days of ink on dead trees, the most authors could expect was perhaps one or two **letters** published, in a leisurely sort of way, several months after their article, to which they might be invited to respond. Now, in the hectic world of electronic publishing, some journals encourage readers to comment, annotate and even rate articles and *PLoS One* goes so far as to describe itself as an interactive journal. If your work has been published in a journal with a rapid response facility, it is a good idea to set up an alert to tell you when comments have been posted. It is also a good idea to agree with your co-authors about how you will respond to such comments.

Since editors find it increasingly difficult to get detailed reviews (because the best qualified people are too busy or can't be bothered), some have suggested that journals should switch from pre- to post-publication review. The idea (which sounds great in theory) is that public-spirited and highly qualified readers would point out flaws in papers and authors could respond by revising their papers. A couple of journals have experimented with this system but found it unworkable, as few readers posted any comments and those that did weren't particularly helpful.

Wager E (2009) If comment is cheap, why is peer review so expensive? (BMJ Blog) http://blogs. bmj.com/bmj/2009/04/16/

Nature peer review trial (2006) *Nature* **442**: xiii doi:10.1038/7099xiiid

■ Press conferences

If you (or your company or institution) want to hold a press conference to announce a publication you must let the journal know. Most editors are delighted by opportunities to publicise work appearing in their journals but you should always liaise closely with the journal or publisher's press department.

Major meetings sometimes invite authors to attend press conferences to talk about their presentations. This can cause problems if your work has already been accepted by a journal with a strict embargo policy, so always check with the journal before agreeing.

See also the sections on **media relations** and **press releases**.

■ Press releases

A press release about research is fine if you issue it in consultation with a journal or meeting but potentially hazardous to the health of your publication if you issue it independently. Journal editors do not like authors talking to the press before an article is published and they particularly dislike results being discussed in newspapers, or on the radio or television, before they appear in the peer-reviewed literature. However, these same editors are delighted by media attention when papers are published. The rule for authors is simple: once your paper has been accepted for publication, do not contact the press without agreement from the journal.

Press interest in meeting presentations can cause problems since this takes place before the full version is published and could, in theory, jeopardise full publication if mishandled. However, most journals appreciate that journalists attend major meetings and accept that preliminary findings may therefore get reported. The general rule is that, if you are questioned by the press, you should provide no more detail than appears in the abstract, since this is already in the public domain. You should not provide copies of slides, the wording of your talk, or extended abstracts. To be on the safe side, you probably should not provide copies of posters to journalists, since these can contain considerable detail. This might seem odd, since attendees at the meeting can see your poster, and you can hand out copies, so you might consider it to be as much in the public domain as the abstract. However, to avoid detailed reports appearing in the press and jeopardising your chance of full publication in a peer-reviewed journal, this is usually the best strategy.

Perhaps surprisingly, most journals do not consider a 'webcast' from a meeting to constitute prior publication.[1]

1 For example: Kassirer JP (1999) Posting presentations at medical meetings on the internet. *NEJM*. **340**: 803.

■ Pre-prints; *see prior publication*

■ Pre-submission enquiries

Some editors welcome pre-submission enquiries from authors seeking guidance about whether their journal is the right place for a particular piece of work or type of publication. If a journal website offers this facility, give it a try but if it does not you may simply be told to submit your article in the usual way and wait for a response. Pre-submission enquiries are especially helpful if you want to submit something that the journal generally commissions (such as an editorial, commentary or book review) or if you are planning something that does not fit into the normal publication categories or is not the type of thing that the journal normally publishes (e.g. a meeting report or guidelines).

A few journals (notably *PLoS Medicine*) require all authors to submit a covering letter and abstract before going on to a full submission. However, other journals work differently. The *BMJ* notes 'it isn't always possible for us to answer every emailed presubmission inquiry' so they have produced a checklist to help authors decide whether the *BMJ* is the right place for their work (which a well-placed informant tells me is known as the 'reject-your-own-paper' system).

■ Primary publication

If a single study produces several publications they are usually classified into primary and secondary. The primary publication is the one that presents the main findings of the study in full for the first time. Primary publications usually follow the **Introduction, Methods, Results and Discussion (IMRAD)** structure and report the study's primary endpoint(s). There might be more than one primary publication (e.g. presenting clinical and economic aspects of a trial) but this is unusual. Since the primary publication should include a detailed description of the research methods, and since readers will need to understand the methods in order to evaluate the findings, having a single paper, or linked papers in the same journal issue, will avoid duplication. If you are developing more than one paper from a single piece of research you should indicate this when you submit any of the papers for publication. It is good practice to include copies of related papers (or manuscripts) in your submission package to reassure the editor that there is not too much overlap or redundancy. Linked papers should be clearly cross-referenced.

Secondary publications (e.g. sub-group analyses and follow-up studies) should not appear before the primary publication and should always reference it. Your publication strategy should take this into account, especially if you plan to publish your primary paper in a prestigious journal with long acceptance and/or **lead times** and a secondary paper in a lower-tier journal that happens to be more rapid.

It is important to distinguish primary from secondary publications to avoid 'double-counting' in reviews and meta-analyses. For example, if data from an interim analysis, six-month follow-up and five-year follow up are published without clear study identification or cross-referencing, the same patients could be included up to three times in a meta-analysis. Since the population characteristics (number of patients, mean age, etc.) will, by definition, differ for each analysis, it can be surprisingly difficult to determine whether the papers report the same study. Including a trial registration number should help reduce confusion when several papers report findings from the same study. To avoid 'double-counting' it is also important to cross-reference **translations** of primary papers clearly to the original publication.

■ Prior publication

Most peer-reviewed journals will consider only work that has not previously been published in full. Some ask authors to state this in their covering letter or to sign a declaration that this is the case. If you want to get your work published, you therefore need to avoid the pitfall of 'prior publication'. The **International Committee of Medical Journal Editors' (ICMJE)** guidelines available at www.icmje.org provide some useful definitions.

In simple terms, **abstracts**, **posters** and **oral presentations** do not constitute prior publication. However, extended abstracts (> 500 words) or conference proceedings sometimes do.

Presenting results at internal (company or institution) meetings, or to investigators or regulators should not affect later publication. However, circulating a research report to a wide audience not involved with the study might cause problems.

Posting reports on websites is currently a grey area. Some journals consider that this is analogous to presenting findings at a meeting, and are not bothered by the appearance of so-called pre-prints.[1] Others take a much firmer line and consider them to be prior publications. Disciplines outside medicine (notably physics) have used pre-print servers for some time and these seem to exist happily alongside the peer-reviewed journals.

Since September 2008, US law has required that results of trials of new drugs that will be sold in the USA must be posted on **ClinicalTrials.gov** under the **FDAAA** legislation. This initially caused concern about whether such postings would constitute **prior publication** (and therefore prevent later publication in a peer-reviewed journal). However, the **ICMJE** announced that posting the summary tables required by FDAAA would not affect publication in a journal; however, they have warned that more extensive release of results via other websites might.

Some journals ask authors to list previous presentations at meetings. This might help readers trying to link abstracts with full papers, which can sometimes be surprisingly tricky. For more on this subject, *see* **trial identification**.

1 For example: Delamothe T, Smith R, Keller MA *et al.* (1999) Netprints: the next phase in the evolution of biomedical publishing. *BMJ.* **319**: 1515–16.

And *see* http://clinmed.netprints.org

2 *BMJ* (2004) News item: drug company to make its trial results public. *BMJ.* **329**: 366.

Wager E and Abbasi K (2008) Medical editors and trial reporting: a betrayal of patient care. *JRSM.* **101**: 4–5.

Marusić A (2008) Registration of clinical trials still moving ahead – September 2008 update to uniform requirements for manuscripts submitted to biomedical journals. *Croat Med J.* **49**: 582–5.

■ Proofs (page proofs)

Journals send (or e-mail) proofs to the corresponding author shortly before publication and often expect these to be checked and returned in a short space of time. For most articles you will receive page proofs, i.e. laid out as the pages will appear in the journal, with figures correctly placed, headers and footers according to journal style, etc. **Galley proofs** (i.e. single columns of text not made up into pages) are almost obsolete except for letters or 'filler' items which get squeezed into issues just before publication.

To prevent delays it is important that the **corresponding author** can be reached and can respond quickly. Although some people believe that the corresponding author indicates some level of merit or seniority (perhaps equating it with the **guarantor**) in practical terms it makes sense to select the person who is most likely to check the proofs efficiently.

Use of conventional proofreading symbols will increase the chances that corrections will be made as you intended. You can find proof-reading marks at:

http://www.journalismcareers.com/articles/proofreadingsymbols.shtml

When reading proofs remember that your article will probably have been put into the journal's **house style**. There is no point in resisting such changes. However, if a copy-editor has changed your meaning or introduced errors, you may correct this. If you discover major problems with the proofs it is best to call the journal to discuss them.

The corresponding author should agree with the other authors, in advance, how the proofs will be handled. There may not be time (or it may not achieve much) to circulate proofs to all authors but, if possible, proofs should be checked by at least two people. Proofreading is when **nitpickers** can be really useful as they often spot mistakes that others miss.

■ Protocol review

Some journals review and publish research protocols before studies are completed. However, this practice has not been widely adopted so if you want your protocol reviewed this may limit your choice of **target journals**. Protocol review has several advantages for researchers. Journals that review protocols sometimes guarantee to publish the findings if the study is completed satisfactorily or at least guarantee that it will undergo external review rather than being rejected after only in-house review. Alternatively, if your protocol is rejected you know there is no point in submitting the results to that journal. If a reviewer spots a flaw in your study design it may not be too late to rectify it. Lastly, publication of the protocol might alert potential participants to the study, which could assist recruitment.

From the journal's (and readers') viewpoint, protocol review offers perhaps the most impartial method of scrutinising a study's design, since the reviewer cannot be influenced by the findings. Publishing the protocol may also prevent **data dredging** or authors presenting *post hoc* analyses as if they were planned.

Some journals (e.g. *BMJ*, *The Lancet* and *PLoS Medicine*) require a copy of the protocol to be submitted with any paper reporting a clinical trial.

Godlee F (2001) Publishing study protocols: making them visible will improve registration, reporting and recruitment. *BMC News and Views*. **2**: 4. http://www.biomedcentral.com/1471-8219/2/4

■ Publication agreements

Agreeing plans for a publication in writing, as early as possible, can avoid much misunderstanding and wrangling later. **GPP2** recommends that publication agreements for company-sponsored studies should be drawn up when the protocol is finalised and that agreements for all other types of company-sponsored publications should be signed before any writing begins.

Agreements for trials should confirm that investigators will have access to the data and will be free to publish the results. The guidelines also recommend that sponsor companies should provide authors with a copy of their **publication policy**. GPP2 also recommends that the agreement should confirm authors' responsibilities to avoid premature or duplicate publication, to disclose conflicts of interest, identify funding sources and ensure authorship is appropriately attributed.

See Appendix 3 (pp. 150–66) for further details.

■ Publication bias

Publication bias occurs when studies with unfavourable findings (either in terms of the sponsor's product or the investigator's pet theory) or those with equivocal results are less likely to be published than those with favourable or positive results. Such bias is further emphasised when positive studies get published more than once, creating **redundant publications**. Some cases of non-publication and covert redundant publication have been well-publicised and have resulted in bad publicity for the perpetrators.

Publication bias can skew the results of systematic reviews and meta-analyses. For this reason, such reviews sometimes include an estimate of publication bias e.g. a funnel plot.

Various strategies to prevent or reduce publication bias have been discussed by journal editors. One is the requirement to register all trials at their inception. In September 2004 the members of the **International Committee of Medical Journal Editors (ICMJE)** announced that **trial registration** would be a requirement for publication in their journals from July 2005. Another initiative is to encourage the inclusion of **trial identifiers** in all publications (e.g. registration or protocol number). The latest version of the Declaration of Helsinki also calls on doctors to publish the results of all research, regardless of whether they are positive or negative.

A well-planned publication strategy should prevent publication bias by ensuring that all studies get published and that redundant publications are not created.

Chalmers I (1990) Underreporting research is scientific misconduct. *JAMA*. **263**: 1405–8.

Melander H, Ahlqvist-Rastad J, Meijer G *et al*. (2003) Evidence b(i)ased medicine – selective reporting from studies sponsored by pharmaceutical industry: review of studies in new drug applications. *BMJ*. **326**: 1171–3.

Tramèr MR, Reynolds DJM, Moore RA *et al*. (1997) Impact of covert duplicate publication on meta-analysis: a case study. *BMJ*. **315**: 635–40.

■ Publication Plan, The

A really useful free website set up in 2008 providing information and news for people involved with publication planning. Definitely worth a look.

www.thepublicationplan.com

■ Publication policy

Any organisation that gets involved with publications ought to have a publication policy. This should set out general principles and reflect relevant guidelines (such as those from the **ICMJE** and **GPP**). Policies, unlike detailed publication strategies, can be public documents, should be applied in all cases and should only need updating when external guidelines change or new issues arise. In contrast, publication strategies and plans are usually internal documents relating to one product or project and require constant updating to reflect the progress of publications.

Helpful policies will include enough detail to inform decisions and avoid platitudes and meaningless management-speak such as 'Heavenly Pharmaceuticals will pro-actively engage in responsible publication practices that will advance the cause of science' (which doesn't really tell you anything).

Publication policies should cover topics such as authorship criteria, data ownership and access, managing and disclosing conflicts of interest as well as general statements about what will be published (e.g. a commitment to publish results of all clinical trials in peer-reviewed journals).

■ Publication steering committee

This is usually just a posh term for a **writing group**. However, for big projects that will generate many publications, it can be helpful to have an overall steering committee to oversee the planning and strategy while each publication will have its own writing group.

Some drug companies appoint a publication steering committee for each product or major trial. This group takes strategic decisions such as how many publications to develop, where to present and publish them, and who the authors should be. The committee is mainly or exclusively comprised of non-company personnel. Each publication then has its own writing group, which includes all the named authors and often several company employees (e.g. statisticians and medical writers).

GPP2 notes that publication steering committees should be formed early in the life of a study (e.g. when the protocol is finalised or at the end of patient recruitment) and that all investigators should be informed about the committee's membership and responsibilities. *See* Appendix 3 (pp. 150–66) for further details.

■ Publication strategy

If you produce a publication strategy document it should fit neatly between your organisation's publication policy and detailed plans for individual publications. However, if you are only dealing with a few publications you might prefer to combine the latter two into a strategic plan – but don't forget that even the simplest publication will work better if you do have a strategy. It can also be easier to get agreement among authors if you start by discussing the strategy in general terms and then consider the details in the plan. Since strategies and plans can merge, there is sometimes confusion about the differences so the following table sets out some general rules.

	Publication policy	*Publication strategy*	*Publication plan*
Applies to	All situations (no exceptions)	A group of publications (and may be revised)	One or more publications (and is frequently revised)
Document is usually	External	Internal – but shared with key people	Internal
Needs updating	Every few years / if external guidelines change	If strategy changes or new data become available	Frequently (to reflect progress of publications)
Refers to / consistent with	External guidelines (e.g. ICMJE)	Internal strategies (e.g. marketing plans)	Publication strategy

For example, the publication policy might state that the company will endeavour to publish results of all clinical trials in peer-reviewed journals. The strategy for a particular study might be to publish one primary paper in a general medical journal and a sub-group analysis in a specialist European gastroenterology journal. The plan would set out the key messages for each paper, the proposed authors, the target audience, the target journal, back-up journals and target dates for publication milestones.

See Chapters 1–3 for more details.

■ Public Library of Science (PLoS)

PLoS describes itself as 'a non-profit organization of scientists and physicians committed to making the world's scientific and medical literature a public resource'. It receives funding from various charities and funds. PLoS launched an electronic medical journal in October 2004. This employs the Open Access model in which content is freely available on the internet, funded by page charges. *PLoS Medicine* has now been joined by *PLoS One*, which has some innovative features such as article-level **metrics** and reader comments and ratings. *See* www.plos.org

■ PubMed

A website run by the US National Library of Medicine which gives access to **Medline** and **PubMed Central**. A useful (and free) resource for searching the literature, checking **MeSH** headings for **key words** and finding out whether a journal is included in **Medline**. The address is: http://www.ncbi.nlm.nih.gov/PubMed

■ PubMed Central

An electronic archive of full-text journal articles launched by the US National Library of Medicine in 2000. Articles include those from fully **Open Access** journals and others from conventional publishers that release research papers after a set period (usually six to 24 months after publication). It can be searched via the PubMed website (which also gives access to **Medline**) http://www.ncbi.nlm.nih.gov/pmc/index.html

Not to be confused with **BioMed Central** which is a commercial company (now part of Springer) that publishes a range of Open Access journals, all of which are available on PubMed Central.

Q

■ Queries

It may seem obvious, but getting a prompt and helpful answer to a query depends on addressing it to the right person or department. Unfortunately, journal functions are often divided between different organisations and companies, so this is not always as straightforward as it might seem. Check the title page or website for contact telephone numbers and e-mail addresses, and to try to unravel who does what. Large, independent journals (like the **'Big Five'**) tend to organise everything under one roof, journals edited by academics and produced by publishers on behalf of academic societies often work out of several locations and can therefore be harder to pin down.

Use the following table as a guide to where you should direct your queries.

Query about	Large, independent journals	Smaller, 'academic' journals
Receipt of manuscript	Editorial department	The Editor/where you submitted the manuscript
When to expect decision	Editorial department	The Editor/where you submitted the manuscript
Appealing a decision	The Editor	The Editor
Serious complaint	The Editor, then **Ombudsman** (if there is one) or Editor's employer	The Editor, then the parent organisation/academic society
When to expect proofs	Journal's Production Department/Assistant Editor assigned to manuscript	Production Department (Publisher)

Query about	Large, independent journals	Smaller, 'academic' journals
Query on proofs	Journal's Production Department/Assistant Editor assigned to manuscript/Technical Editor	Production Department (Publisher)
Ordering offprints/ reprints	Reprint Department	Publisher/Reprint Department
Permission to reproduce figure* etc.	Journal's permissions Department/Publisher	Permissions Department (Publisher)
Readership	Journal's Advertising Department	Advertising Department (Publisher)

*Note: If the original was published in an Open Access journal under a creative commons licence you do not need permission to re-use it, but always check the journal's website.

■ Queues

Printed journals that operate within a strict **page budget** can publish only a certain number of papers in each issue. If the editor accepts more papers than the journal can publish, a queue will form. This explains the lengthy **lead time** between acceptance and publication for some journals (over a year in some cases). If speed of publication is important to you, try to discover the lead time of your **target journal**. If you simply want to cite your publication, then speed of decision may be more important (since you can cite an article as 'in press' once it is accepted). If you need **offprints** by a certain date (e.g. for a particular event), contact the journal for details of their production schedule and to see if you can negotiate something to meet your needs.

Some journals make accepted material available online before it appears in print, but there may still be some delay between acceptance and electronic publication to allow for **technical editing**.

R

■ Readership

See also **target audience**. The best place to get detailed information about the readership of a journal that carries advertisements is the **advertising department** because they use this information to persuade companies to advertise in their journal.

■ Redundant publication

The **International Committee of Medical Journal Editors (ICMJE)** defines redundant publication as anything that overlaps substantially with another publication. The term 'duplicate publication' is sometimes used synonymously, but this may not be strictly accurate, since perpetrators do not necessarily limit themselves to only two publications and the publications may not be exact duplicates. Strict word limits in some journals, or the desire to increase one's publication list, may tempt authors to split their findings into several papers; extreme cases are condemned as **salami slicing**. However, such multiple publication may be acceptable if different parts of the study are understandable by themselves and relevant to different audiences. Some journals offer guidance on how much overlap is acceptable, but this is a grey area. The *BMJ* notes that 'Whenever an article . . . overlaps by more than 10% with previously published work, or work submitted elsewhere, we expect authors to send us copies of those articles'.

Journal editors frown on redundant publication because they prefer to publish original, rather than recycled, material. They may also be concerned that undetected duplication may skew the results of systematic reviews and meta-analyses. The key to preventing such **publication bias** is clear **trial identification**. Secondary analyses, follow-up studies and **translations** should be clearly labelled as such and should always include a reference to the original study.

Companies that have invested heavily in a major study will, understandably, want to get the most out of publications if the findings are favourable. (Although, interestingly, a survey of duplicate publications found that only 33% were sponsored by the pharmaceutical industry, so perhaps academic pressures create an even greater temptation.[1]) However, a responsible publication strategy should not include any redundant publications. If the moral argument is not enough, remember that detection of deliberate redundant publication can bring negative publicity and duplicate articles may be retracted (*see* references for examples). Worse still, almost 70% of journal editors said they would impose restrictions on future submissions for any author found guilty of redundant publication.[2]

1 von Elm E, Poglia G, Walder B *et al.* (2004) Different patterns of duplicate publication: an analysis of articles used in systematic reviews. *JAMA.* **291**: 974–80.

2 Yank V and Barnes D (2003) Consensus and contention regarding redundant publications in clinical research: cross-sectional survey of editors and authors. *J Med Ethics.* **29**: 109–14.

Huston P and Moher D (1996) Redundancy, disaggregation, and the integrity of medical research. *The Lancet.* **347**: 1024–6.

Tramèr MR, Reynolds DJM, Moore RA *et al.* (1997) Impact of covert duplicate publication on meta-analysis: a case study. *BMJ.* **315**: 635–40.

Horton R (2008) Retraction. *The Lancet.* **371**: 288.

■ References

Preparing references can be a tedious job and numerous studies show that reference lists frequently contain errors. One common cause is copying citations from other papers without reading the actual reference. Although it still falls short of perfection, you should at least obtain an abstract and check the reference from **Medline** or the journal website. The best way to overcome the drudgery of typing references and reformatting them is to invest in bibliographic software such as Reference Manager or EndNote.

Even if you have prepared the reference list with great care, it is easy to omit a detail or make a typing mistake. Queries about references tend to be spotted by technical editors rather than reviewers and therefore come at the proof stage, when you are in a hurry and facing a deadline. It is a good habit to take a copy of the first page of every reference cited in a paper and file these with the typescript. This will save a lot of frantic scrabbling about (and may therefore avoid delays) if you need to check a reference later. In this electronic age, a computer file of PDFs or scanned copies would serve just as well – but I bet paper is quicker!

■ Reformatting

If your paper is rejected by your **target journal**, you should check the instructions of your **second target journal** and reformat the typescript so that it complies. The reference section is usually the most time-consuming to reformat, unless you have used bibliographic software to create your reference list, in which case this task will be quick and easy. The other section that often needs adjustment is the abstract, since different journals have different requirements for structure and length.

If you do not reformat your submission you may reduce your chance of acceptance because the reviewer or editor may assume that you could not be bothered to meet the journal's requirements, or (rightly) that the paper has been rejected by another journal. The former is probably worse than the latter. Most editors of specialist journals realise that they have higher acceptance rates than prestigious general journals so a previous rejection should not count against you. Some journals even request copies of previous reviews, although I wonder how many authors are honest enough to comply.

■ Rejection

■ Rates

Rejection rates range from just 10% for some **pay journals** to over 90% for prestigious, general journals (such as the **'Big Five'**). If speed of publication is important, you need to select your target journal carefully, since a string of rejections will delay publication as well as denting your morale. However, some journals with high rejection rates have relatively rapid **decision times** because they reject a high proportion of articles after **in-house review**. Many journals publish rejection (or acceptance) rates on their website. Rates may vary for different parts of the journal; for example short reports and research letters may have lower rejection rates than full papers. The best way to avoid rejection (as well as doing brilliant research) is to research your target journal carefully and then to follow its instructions with equal care.

■ Times

Rejection times range from a few days, for some of the ultra-fast **pay journals** and those that employ **in-house review**, to several months. The worst I have experienced is six months. The average time if your paper undergoes external peer review is around three months -- this is a good figure to use for planning. If you have not heard from a journal after three months you should politely enquire to make sure your manuscript has not been lost or forgotten. This may also spur the editor into nudging a tardy reviewer.

Times from submission to rejection tend to be shorter than those from submission to acceptance, especially for journals that reject a sizeable proportion of papers without sending them for external peer review. It may therefore be worth the risk of submitting to a journal with a high **rejection rate** if you can be fairly sure of a rapid rejection. In this case, honour will have been satisfied that you attempted to get into a high **impact factor** or prestigious journal but you will not have wasted too much time in the attempt.

However, on a gloomier note, remember that journals with high rejection rates still reject many papers after sending them out for external peer review and, in some cases, even after asking authors to respond to reviewers' comments. Coming close to acceptance may therefore be a worse fate than a swift, outright rejection, unless the reviewers suggest changes that will increase your chance of acceptance by another journal.

The psychological effects of rejection seem worse if you have waited a long time for a decision and it is easy to lose momentum and motivation. It is therefore vital to have a **back-up plan**.

■ Reprints

Strictly speaking, a reprint is a copy of an article produced after publication. The correct term for extra copies ordered at the time of publication is **offprints** (although the terms are often used interchangeably), so *see* this section for further details.

In the old days receiving reprint (or offprint) requests from far-flung spots was a pleasant by-product of publication and a good way of enhancing your stamp collection. These days, most researchers seem to have access to electronic libraries or photocopiers, so requests are rarer, but still enjoyable. Remember that only the corresponding author will have this pleasure (and collect the stamps), so it is a nice idea to keep other authors informed.

■ Retractions

If a journal discovers that it has published a flawed or misleading paper (either because of honest error or because of scientific misconduct such as plagiarism or fraud) it may retract the paper. The notice of retraction will appear in indexing systems that cover the journal. Although, in complex studies, contributors may take responsibility for only part of the research, all authors (or contributors) will be affected by such a retraction, so think hard before putting your name on a paper if you have any doubts about it. Editors may retract articles for publication misconduct (e.g. **redundant publication)** as well as research fraud.

■ Reviewer choice

Some journals allow authors to suggest potential reviewers. It is hard to discover how often editors act on these suggestions, although journals that require suggestions (such as **BioMed Central)** almost certainly use them more often than those that do not. If your target journal requires reviewer suggestions, discuss potential reviewers with the writing group and agree on your suggestions well before submission (don't leave it to the last minute). Check the journal's criteria, for example people from the same institution and previous co-authors are usually disallowed. Remember that you usually need to supply email addresses for the suggested reviewers.

Authors may also indicate if there is anybody who should be excluded from the review process (e.g. on the grounds of a strong competing interest). Again, it is difficult to know whether editors honour these requests all the time. Cynics have suggested that identifying somebody you think should not review your paper might be counterproductive, as the editor would be tempted to use this person just to ensure a really tough review. Journal editors will probably protest that they are not like that . . . and in fact this was the response I got to an informal survey.[1]

Some electronic submission forms have spaces for proposing or opposing reviewers. If this facility is not available and you feel strongly that an individual should not review your paper, you should mention this in your covering letter. Editors are most likely to respect your wishes if you give a compelling (and polite) explanation, such as an insurmountable conflict of interest. Implying that the individual is mentally unstable or a cantankerous old curmudgeon will probably not advance your cause.

1 Wager E (2004) Use of author-nominated reviewers: an informal survey. *European Science Editing.* 30: 117–8.

Wager E, Parkin EC and Tamber PS (2006) Are reviewers suggested by authors as good as those chosen by editors? Results of a rater-blinded, retrospective study. *BMC Medicine.* **4:** 13.

■ Reviewers' comments

Unconditional acceptances are incredibly rare, so you will nearly always have to respond to reviewers' comments. If your work is rejected and you plan to submit it to another journal you can, of course, ignore these comments but it makes sense to swallow your pride and read them, once your disappointment has worn off, to see if they identify any obvious mistakes or ways in which you could improve your paper. (It is also possible that your second target journal will use the same reviewer as the first – in which case it is definitely preferable to have followed at least some of his or her suggestions.)

If you receive a conditional acceptance you may still need to swallow a little pride but you should consider reviewers' comments as negotiable suggestions rather than a diktat and, if you can provide good reasons, you do not have to follow them all. Hywel Williams (an experienced editor, reviewer and author) notes 'referees are not gods, but human beings who make mistakes', and goes on to suggest three golden rules: 'answer completely, answer politely and answer with evidence'.[1]

Most journals ask authors for a detailed response, either in a covering letter or a list, to show that you have responded to every point. You may also be asked to supply a copy of the paper with revisions highlighted. As well as helping the journal editor, these are useful tools for discussing revisions with co-authors. The **corresponding author** will receive the reviewers' comments, but this does not mean that s/he has to draft the entire response. It is often best to divide the questions among authors depending on their expertise. However you organise the response, make sure to involve all your **key players**, since everybody must approve the final version.

Your response should be polite and professional. Where possible, and especially if you are explaining why you have not made a suggested change, support your argument with evidence (e.g. references) just as you would in a paper. If reviewers request conflicting actions (e.g. to expand and cut the same section) check the editor's covering letter, which should indicate how to handle this, or contact the editor for advice. Do not forget to respond to points in the editor's letter as well as to those in the reviewers' reports. In fact, editors' requests should take priority over reviewer suggestions.

Some journals set a deadline for responding (often four to six weeks). If this causes insurmountable problems (e.g. if you have to perform extra analyses and simply cannot get them done in time) contact the editor as soon as possible to explain the situation and see if you can negotiate an extension. If you plan not to resubmit, it is helpful to let the journal know. However, if possible, try to respond reasonably promptly. Most people find revisions vaguely dispiriting, so it is tempting to postpone this task and its prospect only gets worse the longer you procrastinate. Think positive, congratulate yourself on getting a conditional acceptance (if, indeed, you have) and consider this the penultimate stage towards your publication goal. Or bribe yourself with promises of a stiff drink/chocolate/your favourite legal indulgence once you have resubmitted.

On a gloomier note, read the letter from the editor carefully. Some journals only agree to 'reconsider' your paper after you have responded to the reviewers' comments, and may reject a fair proportion after this stage. (For example, *The Lancet*'s instructions state: 'Submissions that survive in-house and peer review might be referred back to authors for revision. This is an invitation to present the best possible paper for further scrutiny by the journal; it is not an acceptance'.) Receiving a rejection after you have made revisions may seem unfair and annoying, but it is even more irksome if you have gone around telling everybody that your paper has been accepted.

Some journals ask authors to send reviewers' comments they have received from other journals. I used to think this was a rather ridiculous request, as most authors don't want to admit that their work has already been rejected by another journal. However, I am softening my views on this strategy, and even recommending it in some cases, since hearing that some journals will accept a publication on the basis of another journal's review, especially if the reviewers liked the paper but the editor thought it was better suited for a different type of journal. The most obvious example would be if your paper was good enough to be sent out for external review by a really top-notch general journal (like *The Lancet* or *NEJM*) and you are now submitting it to a specialist journal. Supplying reviewers' comments should also prevent a journal from sending your paper to the same reviewer again (but only if the review is signed). If you do pass reviewers' comments from one journal to another, you may also include a rebuttal explaining why you have not made all the suggested changes – but the second editor will probably expect you to have addressed at least some of the issues raised by the reviewers.

1 Williams HC (2004) How to reply to referees' comments when submitting manuscripts for publication. *J Am Acad Dermatol.* **51**: 79–83.

■ Review process

The *BMJ* once included a delightful typo that changed external review into eternal review.[1] This provides a useful mnemonic for the two basic review processes and the effects they have on review speed.

Journals that have high **rejection rates** and employ a substantial editorial staff often reject up to 50% of submissions after **internal review** alone. Only those papers that the editors consider they are likely to publish are sent for review by external experts. This system means that **rejection times** tend to be much shorter than acceptance times (*see* **acceptance times** for details). It may therefore make sense to submit to such a journal even if you harbour only a slim hope of acceptance since rejection is likely to be swift.

Less well-staffed journals (i.e. those edited by academics rather than full-time editors) tend to send all submissions for **external review** and, subsequently, rejection and acceptance take about the same length of time. Journals may either use **editorial board** members or a larger database of reviewers to review papers, but this difference probably has little effect on the time to get a decision. Journals that offer rapid review may pay their reviewers (but that is not the reason these are usually referred to as **pay journals**).

Once the editor has received the reviewers' reports, the submission may be discussed at an editorial board or selection committee meeting, e.g. the *BMJ*'s **Hanging Committee**. If meetings are infrequent, this may increase the time to get a decision. Further delay may be caused by additional reviews, e.g. by a statistician.

Some journals ask authors to suggest potential reviewers, but (according to an informal survey that I carried out) this does not seem to increase the number of reviews obtained for each paper so it is unlikely to affect the speed of review.

1 Latham JN (2004) Just how rapid is 'eternal' review? *BMJ.* **329**: 801.

■ Running title

This is a short version of a paper's title that often appears as a header on the journal page and is usually written on the title page of a typescript. Check your target journal's instructions to see if a running title is required and, if so, how long it can be. This is one of those minor points which, if you forget it, or fail to follow the instructions, should not really affect your paper's chance of acceptance but which, especially if combined with other minor offences, is likely to annoy editors, perhaps suggest that your paper has been rejected by another journal, and generally give a poor impression. Try to include the running title on an early draft of the paper, since all authors should approve it and it may be overlooked on the pre-submission check. Condensing a title often has the effect of making it more direct, especially if it describes the study findings rather than just the study design. It is therefore important to ensure that it is justified and not over promotional.

S

■ Salami science / slicing

This descriptive phrase, originally coined by Ed Huth, refers to the much frowned-upon practice of splitting or re-analysing data from a single study to generate as many publications as possible.[1] It probably occurs equally in academia (where researchers are judged by the length rather than the quality of their CV) and industry (where companies are keen to get positive findings published as often as possible). As with many questions in scientific publication, good judgement is required when deciding how many publications your findings warrant. In answering this question, try to keep the reader in mind and consider which results should be presented together.

As a general rule, most clinical trials generate a single, primary paper, which describes the primary outcome set out in the protocol and often some of the secondary outcomes or incidental findings. This may, legitimately, be followed by secondary papers describing sub-set analyses or follow-ups. It is common for economic findings to be presented separately from clinical ones; however the *BMJ* will not consider **economic evaluations** on their own.[2]

If you do produce more than one paper from a publication, make sure that the links are transparent (e.g. by including a **trial identifier** or registration number) and always reference the primary publication.

1 Huth EJ (1986) Irresponsible authorship and wasteful publication. *Ann Intern Med*. **104**: 257–9.

2 Smith R (2002) New *BMJ* policy on economic evaluation. *BMJ*. **325**: 1124.

■ Secondary publications

Most studies produce one, fat, juicy publication reporting the main findings – this is termed the **primary publication**. Virtually everything else is considered a secondary publication. The distinction is important because secondary publications should not appear before the primary one and should always reference it. To avoid data from the same study getting included more than once in meta-analyses, it is also good practice to include a trial registration number on all publications, so readers can tell when different papers refer to the same trial.

Secondary publications can include sub-group analyses, follow-up studies and **translations**. Publications that do not present original data, such as review articles, may also be considered secondary publications.

■ Second target journal

Always select a second target journal in case you get rejected by your first target. Try to select the second journal at the same time as the first because you will have all the relevant journal information to hand and you may not get another chance to discuss this face-to-face if you are planning only one or two **meetings (of the writing group)**. If you do not select a second journal at this stage you may delay resubmission by trying to gather opinions. It may also be more difficult to reach agreement when everybody is in a bad mood after the first rejection.

■ Selective publication

Something to avoid: this is the practice of publishing only those studies that favour your product or theory, or of publishing only those parts of a study that are positive. In the first case, it leads to **publication bias**, which can distort the literature and skew meta-analyses. In the second, it produces misleading papers. One remedy for under-publication is **trial registration**, which has been a requirement for papers submitted to journals edited by the **International Committee of Medical Journal Editors (ICMJE)** committee members since July 2005. If a journal suspects selective publication of results, it may request a copy of the protocol. Many journals reserve the right to do this, and a few (e.g. *The Lancet* and **PLoS**) require protocols to be submitted routinely.

Even if your intentions are honourable, you will sometimes have to decide which findings to omit from a short paper. One solution to the problem of presenting a large dataset within a stringent word limit is to publish **supplementary material** on the journal's website. Another solution is to produce more than one paper, but you should avoid **salami slicing**.

■ Short reports

In the olden days of ink and dead trees, parsimonious editors guarded their precious pages fiercely and encouraged short publications. This meant that short reports or research letters generally had higher acceptance rates than full-length articles. Now in the magical era of electronic publishing, the rules have changed. Some journals publish long web versions and shorter printed ones (*see* **ELPS**) so the truly short report may be on the verge of extinction. However some old-fashioned journals whose print and web versions are identical may still include different formats and they are worth considering.

■ Short title; *see* running title

■ Slides

Slides are often used to illustrate **oral presentations** at meetings, but organisers rarely provide guidance about how to prepare them. If you do not have much experience of giving talks at conferences, or if the prospect worries you, consult friendly colleagues and/or books.

You should not give copies of your slides to journalists since this could lead to extensive reporting which might jeopardise full publication in a journal. However, you may provide your abstract since this is considered to be in the public domain. Although journals may permit webcasts from conferences, they may be less happy if a company or institution posts slides on its website before publication, so it is best to avoid this.

When working with co-authors or sponsors, ensure there is enough time for everybody to comment on the presentation. You will probably be allowed to talk for only about ten minutes, so it is crucial to focus on your **key message** and decide what you are going to leave out. Unlike papers, graphs are often better than complex tables at conveying messages on slides.

Fraser J and Cave R (2004) *Presenting in Biomedicine: 500 tips for success*. Radcliffe Publishing, Oxford.

Hall GM (ed.) (2001) *How to Present at Meetings*. BMJ Books, London.

■ Strategy

This term comes from the Greek word for army (*stratos*) and the verb to lead (*ago*). Although the mental image of warfare is perhaps unfortunate, it does remind us that lots of people are usually involved in publications, and that good leadership and communication are vital. However, unlike an army, there is rarely a single leader who can bark orders at the others and demand undying loyalty. A successful leader in terms of publications is someone who can guide the group with sound knowledge and facilitate decision making.

In both warfare and publications, it is important to have clear objectives and to ensure that these are shared by all members of the group (*see* **expectations** for more about this). A good strategy therefore starts with a clear agreement on what you want to achieve, for example presentations at international anaesthetics meetings in autumn 2012 and a full paper published in a respected, peer-reviewed anaesthetics journal by summer 2013. Once you have agreed the objective you can move on to your tactics, or plan (*see* Chapter 2 'Developing a publication plan . . .' (pp. 7–12)). This will involve choice of target meetings and journal, sorting out **authorship** and agreeing a detailed timetable for who does what.

If you are planning several publications from one piece of research (e.g. a couple of abstracts, a main paper and a secondary publication) it is important to plan them together to ensure a coherent strategy.

■ STROBE

Guidelines for Strengthening The Reporting of OBservational studies in Epidemiology which have been endorsed by many journals. Like **CONSORT**, these guidelines include a checklist, which you need to include when submitting to some journals. However, as the guidelines are more recent than CONSORT, not so many journals insist on this, but it certainly won't do any harm to use it.

www.strobe-statement.org

■ Style

If you are fanatical about writing style, and consider your own to be matchless, you should limit your writing to single-author works, which, these days, usually means editorials, reviews and books. Most research involves collaboration, and, while papers should not be written by committee, they should represent a team effort, which means that strong personal styles are out of place. The writer's style may be further compromised by the journal's **house style**, which is non-negotiable.

If you are preparing a research paper, and particularly if several people are drafting different sections, you should aim for a neutral style. This does not mean that the paper has to be wordy, jargon-ridden or boring, merely that you should curb any tendency to florid prose or personal idiosyncrasies. Once the fragments have been assembled and everybody has agreed on the content it is a good idea for one person to go through the whole paper to make the style as consistent as possible.

If you find the mere thought of writing terrifying, and consider discussions of style to be more appropriate to literature classes or book clubs, take a recent issue of your **target journal** and read three or four papers describing broadly similar research to yours. This should give you a taste of the kind of style the journal prefers. If you cannot find papers describing research broadly similar to yours, you may have selected the wrong journal (in which case, read the section on **journal choice** again). Do not copy chunks of other papers, or try to follow their style too slavishly, but, if you are unsure how much detail to include, or get stuck trying to phrase something, it may help to re-read these papers when you are writing.

Your submission does not need to look exactly like the final journal page – this is the job of the technical editor and typesetter (*see* **house style**). However, you need to follow the instructions and ensure major features are correct, in particular the style for references. Submitting a paper styled for another journal creates a poor impression of carelessness or suspicions that it has already been rejected by another journal.

If you want to improve your writing style read:

Strunk W and White EB (1979) *The Elements of Style* (3e). Allyn & Bacon, Massachusetts. Also available at www.bartleby.com/141/

■ Sub-editing; *see* technical editing

■ Submission letter; *see* covering letter

■ Supplementary material

Some journals publish short versions in the paper edition but permit (or even encourage) longer versions, or the provision of supplementary material, on their website. The *BMJ* refers to this principle as Electronic Long, Paper Short (or **ELPS**). If you have a very rich dataset, or information in a format unsuitable for print, such as extensive colour images, video clips or massive tables, you should check for this facility when choosing your target journal.

Check what formats the journal can accept, and at what stage. For example, you may not be able to submit video clips at the initial reviewing stage, but you should mention that they are available in your covering letter. Whenever possible, try to stick to word limits, and make it clear which material you would be prepared to consider supplementary to the print version (i.e. which may appear only on the website).

If you want to cite supplementary information, give the precise web address and the date you accessed it. Some journals assign special identifiers to electronic material or link electronic components to the paper version using the **DOI (Digital Object Identifier) system**.

■ Supplements

Some journals publish supplements, which are funded by a sponsor and usually cover a specific theme or present the proceedings of a meeting. Such sponsored supplements can be useful vehicles for publishing articles that might be of insufficient interest to be published in the parent journal. However, most journals will not accept papers that are of lower quality than those they normally publish. This was clearly not always the case, since a 1994 study showed that many readers' scepticism about material published in supplements was well founded.[1]

Most journals now state that supplements undergo similar peer review to the parent journal. However, this review is probably directed more to the scientific merit of the articles than to whether they are of interest to readers. Supplements have traditionally been used to repackage or collate several studies, for example to bring together preclinical research about a new drug. This can help readers who might not have access to the original work published in obscure journals. However, a supplement should not be viewed as a licence to create **redundant publication**, and secondary papers should clearly reference their primary sources.

If a supplement is used to present the proceedings of a meeting, you need to ensure that all presenters are happy for their work to appear in this form. There is no rule that new data should not be published in supplements, but this will preclude publication in another journal and may not be the author's first choice. References to supplements usually include the supplement number and may use a different page numbering system from the parent journal (e.g. Vol. 14 (Suppl. 1): S17–32), making it clear to sharp-eyed readers that they did not appear in the main journal. Given the slightly tarnished reputation of supplements, it is usually a better strategy to publish primary papers elsewhere.

Some journals insist that supplements are edited by somebody from outside the sponsoring organisation (although this does not preclude professional writing assistance).

If you are considering a supplement, first check that your target journal actually produces these, and then contact the journal to discover how it handles them. You will need to find out how material is reviewed (and how long this will take), what the costs are, and if there are any special requirements, such as having an independent editor.

1 Rochon P, Gurwitz JH, Cheung CM *et al.* (1994) Evaluating the quality of articles published in journal supplements compared with the quality of those published in the parent journal. *JAMA.* **272**: 108–13.

T

■ Tables

Deciding which data are best presented in tables is an important aspect of planning a paper. Most journals do not allow data to be repeated in text, tables and **figures**, so you need to choose the best format. Remember that a table should normally include at least two columns of figures – most journals will not accept tables with only one column of data, as this can easily be expressed as a list (which takes up less space). However, single-column tables are acceptable for posters. Some congresses allow small tables in abstracts, and this can be a good way to present results, but check the congress requirements since many do not.

You should start planning the tables when the **data analysis plan** is being developed to ensure that the statistical report provides the information you need for the publication.

When preparing a paper, keep tables separate from the text, at the end of the paper. Even if they look inelegant and spill on to more than one page, manuscript tables should always be double-spaced. If you are preparing a disk or submitting a paper electronically use the table function or tabs on your word processing software – do not separate columns using simple word spacing as the data are likely to get garbled. Most journal tables do not include vertical lines to separate columns, so you should avoid using these. Even if you have submitted an electronic version of your manuscript, pay particular attention to tables in the proofs, as numbers often get displaced. The best way to proofread a complex table is to ask a colleague to read out the numbers from the original version while you check the proof.

For more information about tables try Chapter 14 in:

Huth EJ (1999) *Writing and Publishing in Medicine* (3e). Williams & Wilkins, Baltimore.

■ Target audience

Identifying your readers is an important step in planning any publication since it should influence your choice of meeting and journal and the way in which you present the findings. To identify your target audience, think hard about who might actually be interested in your findings rather than who you think ought to be interested. (This is sometimes called the 'Who cares?' test.) Consider not only who your ideal readers are (e.g. haematologists) but where they work (e.g. Europe) and how advanced they are in their specialty (e.g. consultants).

Identifying the target audience for each publication is not only a key part of the publication strategy, but also helps to focus the writing and determine the **key message**. If the authors are not members of the target audience (e.g. specialists writing for generalists) try to include somebody from the target audience in your **internal review**.

■ Target journal

Agree on the journal to which you will submit your paper (i.e. your target) as early as possible. Writing a paper before you have defined your target journal can be a waste of time because it indicates that you have not really considered your **target audience** and it also means you will have to go back and check requirements for length, style and format. *See also* **journal choice** for more details.

■ Technical editing

This may be considered the final stage of the peer-review process (unless one counts **post-publication** comments). Technical editing (also called copy editing or sub-editing) involves checking the submission carefully, correcting or improving the language and putting it into the journal's **house style**. Major journals usually employ (or hire) professional copy editors. Although such copy editors lack specialist qualifications most are skilled at spotting inconsistencies and errors that expert reviewers and authors fail to notice. In some smaller journals, the job of technical editing falls to the editor or members of the **editorial board**.

The amount of technical editing that your paper undergoes will depend on the journal. Some (e.g. the **'Big Five'** and many traditional specialty journals) invest heavily in this; others (mostly the newer, electronic journals) hardly at all. You can judge the degree of technical editing practised by a journal by perusing back issues. If all articles not only have a clear house style in terms of spelling (e.g. US or UK), abbreviations and layout, but also have a certain uniformity of prose style, they are likely to have been heavily edited. If you are submitting to a journal that does minimal copy editing you might choose to get a professional copy editor, or a colleague with a talent for this sort of thing, to check your proofs.

If your work has been heavily edited there is little you can (or should) do about this, unless the editing has introduced ambiguity or changed your meaning, in which case you should politely point this out and correct the problem on the proofs. However, if the copy editor changes your meaning, resist the urge simply to change the text back to the original, since, if the copy editor did not understand you, there is a good chance that some readers will have the same problem, so it makes sense to try to find an alternative wording.

There is some evidence that technical editing improves the readability of papers.[1] However, many people who enjoy writing and have developed a strong personal style dislike having that **style** diluted and their 'voice' removed.

1 Wager E and Middleton P (2002) Effects of technical editing in biomedical journals: a systematic review. *JAMA*. **287**: 2821–4.

■ The International Publication Planning Association (TIPPA)

Run by a commercial conference company, TIPPA is much less of an active membership organisation than **ISMPP** but it does hold interesting meetings, usually in the USA. These are a good chance to meet others involved in publication planning and hear about recent developments.

www.publicationplanningassociation.org

■ The Publication Plan; *see* Publication Plan, The

■ 'Throwaways'; *see* freebies; pay journals

■ Timing

So many factors can affect the timing of a publication that it is impossible to summarise in a short entry. Consult Chapter 3 'How long will it take?' (pp. 13–16) for more details but remember that best case scenarios are rare occurrences, humans are fallible, most people involved in developing publications have chronically over-filled diaries, and we all know what happens to the 'best laid plans of mice and men . . .' although, I have to admit that I have never yet come across a mouse who was planning to publish any research.

■ Title

■ Papers and abstracts

Take care composing the title of your publications, since a good title can attract readers, while a poor one may be the only section they read. Check the requirements of your target meeting or journal. Conferences sometimes limit the length of abstract titles, while some journals specify what you should, or should not, include. In general, you should avoid abbreviations, unless they are universally understood (such as DNA). You should also avoid using drug trade names, since many journals forbid their use in the title, and brand names often differ from country to country, so it is best to use the generic name. Use of the trade name in the title may also give your publication an unduly commercial feel and prejudice some reviewers and readers.

Creating a good title is a balancing act between including all the pertinent information and keeping it short. In your efforts to restrict the number of words avoid 'noun strings' which can be hard to read. A noun string occurs when too many nouns act as adjectives, for example: 'Oral iron supplementation induced intestinal oxidative stress'. Although it takes a few more words, it is clearer to write: 'Intestinal oxidative stress induced by oral iron supplementation'.

Aim to begin with important words, which will interest the reader, and put details such as the trial design at the end (otherwise most titles will begin 'A randomised, controlled study of . . .'). Check your target journal for its **house style** regarding punctuation or subtitles (e.g. the *BMJ* has a fondness for colons, so you will often see the format 'X versus Y in dread disease: a randomised, controlled trial'). Including details of the trial design in the title may increase your chance of the publication being correctly indexed and therefore retrieved by researchers.

While brand names should be avoided, trial names can be useful since they identify related publications. However, ingenious acronyms for trials have become so fashionable that there is a slight risk that you will pick an acronym already used by another study, and thus cause confusion. For this reason use of a less exciting **trial identifier**, such as a protocol number or **trial registration** number, may be better.

Some journals allow declarative (or informative) titles, which describe your results, for example: 'Wunderdrug improves glycaemic control in type II diabetes'. However, many journals permit only descriptive (or indicative) titles which describe the study but not the results, for example 'Glycaemic control in type II diabetes: a randomised, placebo-controlled trial of Wunderdrug'.

When writing the title for an **abstract**, remember you will have to use the same title if you present as a **poster**, so think about how it looks and whether it will stand out from the crowd. Questions and short titles may be more effective at grabbing attention than the detailed titles often used for journal articles.

Good titles arouse potential readers' curiosity without being opaque or baffling. You can be more creative with titles for editorials and reviews than for trial reports, but remember that your audience may not share a common culture, so references to your favourite pop song, television series or children's book may confuse many readers. Titles that pose a question or conjure up a strong mental image can grab readers' attention – I once entitled a rather dull essay on regulations governing doctors' relations with drug companies, 'How to dance with porcupines', and was pleasantly surprised how much positive feedback I got.

■ Journals

Do not be fooled by journal titles: they are not always a good indication of a journal's scope or nature. Some journals retain titles that have little bearing on their current contents – for example, the *Philosophical Transactions of the Royal Society (B)* is a respected biology journal dating from the 17th century when natural history was called philosophy. Even recent journals may have undergone a change in emphasis so that their title no longer reflects their content – for example, the *Journal of Experimental Medicine* is about immunology. Others have such mundane titles that it is impossible to guess what will interest them. When assessing possible **target journals** try to get copies of three to six of the most recent issues to determine the scope, accepted formats, **hot topics**, length of articles, etc. If you cannot get actual copies, check the website for contents lists or a sample issue. If that fails, contact the publisher who will usually be prepared to supply a sample copy.

■ Title page

Check the journal's requirements and gather all the information you need for the title page of your submission as early as possible. Get authors to check their details on the first draft they see and do not be tempted to leave this section until just before submission (when you can be sure that at least one author will be uncontactable and you will waste valuable time chasing irritating details).

All journals will require the authors' names (*see* **names** for how to present these), their **affiliation** (now and when they did the work) and full contact details for the corresponding author (including fax and e-mail). Many US journals also require authors' highest degrees.

■ Translations

To make your research accessible to a wide audience you might consider presentations at local meetings and publications in several languages. Local language journals have an important role in reaching clinicians but are often considered less prestigious (and have lower **impact factors**) than English-language journals. Some journals will consider translations of published papers but these must reference the original paper and be faithful to the source (e.g. they should not contain new material). An alternative (and sometimes quicker) solution is to ask the original journal for reprint translations. Major publishers are often happy to provide these (for a fee). If you prepare a new version for a second audience (e.g. with emphasis on local findings) take care that this does not constitute **redundant publication**.

■ Trial identifier

Some trials generate several publications. These can be legitimate, for example a couple of abstracts, a primary paper and a follow-up report or secondary analysis, but they may represent **redundant publication** and contribute to **publication bias**. One simple solution for preventing confusion is to include a trial identifier on all publications. Trial identifiers allow readers to see whether publications are linked (e.g. which full reports relate to previous abstracts or other publications) and removes the risk of inadvertently double-counting trials in meta-analysis. Good Publication Practice (GPP) for pharmaceutical companies recommends that trial identifiers should be included on all publications (*see* Appendix 3 for GPP guidelines).

A trial identifier may simply be the sponsor's protocol number, or may be linked with inclusion in a public trial register (such as the ISRCTN). Since July 2005 members of the **International Committee of Medical Journal Editors (ICMJE)** have required **trial registration** as a condition for publication in their journals.

So far, conference organisers have not come out in support of trial identifiers, and it may be difficult to squeeze this information on to an abstract if space is limited. One possible solution is to refer to the trial name in the title or include a group name in the author list (e.g. Bloggs & Cloggs on behalf of the AQ153 Study Group). However, not all conference websites permit this. Another option is to include the trial identifier within the funding acknowledgement (e.g. this study was funded by the Wunderdrug Corporation, protocol number ZZ123).

Wager E (2004) The need for trial identifiers. *Curr Med Res Opin.* **20**: 203–6.

■ Trial registration

Groups that prepare systematic reviews, such as the Cochrane Collaboration, have long argued that details of all trials should be prospectively entered on to a register so that researchers, and potential participants, can see what trials are taking place or have been completed. In this way, they argue, **publication bias** caused by non-publication of unfavourable findings will be prevented. Various trial registers have been established but until recently they were largely voluntary and did not have much to do with publications. However, in September 2004, the members of the **International Committee of Medical Journal Editors (ICMJE)** announced that trial registration would be a requirement for publication in their journals from July 2005.

(For a list of the ICMJE members, *see* **International Committee of Medical Journal Editors**.) Since then, many other journals have followed the ICMJE's lead in making prospective registration a requirement (i.e. trials must be registered when they start and the registration number must be stated in all publications).

De Angelis C, Drazen JM, Frizelle FA *et al*. (2004) Clinical trial registration: a statement from the International Committee of Medical Journal Editors. *The Lancet*. **364**: 911–12.

U

■ Uniform Requirements

This guide, published by the **International Committee of Medical Journal Editors (ICMJE)**, is the best single source for discovering what journal editors expect from authors and sponsors. It covers topics such as **authorship, conflict of interest** and **redundant publication**. It should be required reading for anybody involved with publication strategy. If you cannot find the answer to your question in your target journal's instructions, try the Uniform Requirements for Submission of Manuscripts to Biomedical Journals (to give it its full name). They are available at www.icmje.org

■ Unpublished data (references to)

If you want to refer to unpublished data you need to be aware of some general rules and of individual journal restrictions on this (since they vary).

Once a paper has been accepted for publication it can be cited as being 'in press'. Such a reference looks the same as any other, with a full list of authors, title and journal details, and, where possible, the expected year of publication, but the journal volume and page numbers are simply replaced by the words 'in press'. Only papers that have been accepted (in full) may be cited as 'in press'. A conditional acceptance (i.e. a statement that the journal will reconsider the paper or might publish if the reviewers' comments can be addressed) does not mean the paper is 'in press' since it is possible that the journal will not publish it. Some journals therefore require a copy of the acceptance letter to establish that an article is truly 'in press' and that the author is not being over-optimistic.

Submitting work to a journal or meeting does not equate to it being 'in press'. This may be frustrating, but consider it from the reader's viewpoint. If a reference lists something as, for example, 'submitted to *The Lancet*' there is a strong chance (>90%) that the paper will be rejected, and will therefore not appear in *The Lancet*. Moreover, when the paper is finally accepted, or sent to another journal, the title (and possibly even the author list) may have changed, so it may be difficult for the reader to locate the reference.

Most journals allow citation of published abstracts and associated presentations at meetings, but some, for example *Circulation*, do not. Such citations usually include the name of the meeting, its location and date, as well as the abstract title and authors' names. If the abstract also appears in a journal you should include its title since readers are more likely to have access to journals than to conference proceedings. For example, abstracts presented at the American Society of Hematology appear in a special edition of the journal *Blood*. Some journals (e.g. *Annals of Internal Medicine*) will only accept references published in journals.

If your **target journal** does not permit you to cite an abstract or presentation you may have to include it as a **personal communication** giving brief details in the text, but nothing in the reference list.

ClinicalTrials.gov gives guidance on how to cite studies in this database. *See* http://www.nlm.nih.gov/services/ctcite/htm

V

■ Vancouver Group

Another name for the **International Committee of Medical Journal Editors (ICJME)** – because they first met in Vancouver.

■ Verbal branding

Verbal branding is a marketing term, but, even if you think your publication has nothing to do with marketing, read on, because you need to understand it if you work with drug companies, and you might even find the concept helpful in non-commercial research. Verbal branding simply means the careful and consistent choice of words.

While it usually applies to a pharmaceutical product, verbal branding can be used to deliver any message consistently and effectively. Good communicators probably use verbal branding instinctively by choosing powerful phrases to get their message across.

Some companies develop preferred terms and phrases for describing their products and their competitors. Preferred language may even extend to the drug's indications, and companies have sometimes been accused of creating or promoting new diseases. However, some new terms are more precise or less stigmatising than traditional ones, so they should not all be dismissed as marketing gimmicks. The company's usual aim is to harmonise product descriptions used in promotional material and in the scientific literature so that publications reinforce marketing messages and strengthen the brand image.

The words used to describe mental illness are a good example of the power of language. Disparaging and insensitive terms such as 'spastic' and 'mentally deficient' have now been replaced by 'cerebral palsy' and 'learning disability'. Similarly, powerful painkillers tend to be called opioids rather than narcotics, because of associations with drug abuse. On the subject of drugs, have you ever noticed how critical articles tend to refer to drug companies, while the firms refer to themselves as the pharmaceutical industry?

If you think that verbal branding will lead to repetitive writing, I can only refer you to Fowler's splendid tirade against what he calls 'elegant variation' (i.e. the mistake of believing you must use different words if you mention something more than once):[1]

> It is the second-rate writers, those intent rather on expressing themselves prettily than on conveying their meaning clearly, and still more those whose notions of style are based on a few misleading rules of thumb, that are chiefly open to the allurements of elegant variation. . . . The fatal influence is the advice given to young writers never to use the same word twice in a sentence – or within 20 lines or other limit.

Remember that, while preferred spellings and formats can be used on internal documents and marketing material, peer-reviewed journals impose their own **house style** on papers, so these details may be changed in the final publication. Also, most journals insist that generic product names should be used in papers, and restrict the use of trade names, which can usually be mentioned only once, in the methods section, and often may not be used in titles. When preparing articles for submission to peer-review journals it is therefore important to follow journal guidelines and to be aware that the journal will impose its house style on the published version.

1   Fowler HW (1965) *A Dictionary of Modern English Usage* (2e). Oxford University Press, Oxford.

■ Veto

Research sponsors, be they commercial companies, charities or public institutions, should not have the right to veto a publication. Researchers should check their **contract** or **publication agreement** carefully to ensure they are free to publish their findings.

Differences of opinion may arise between sponsors and investigators, and also between co-authors. The best way to avoid protracted negotiations from delaying the publication schedule is to involve all interested parties in the earliest stages of planning. Ideally, everybody should meet to discuss the findings and agree the publication strategy. If a meeting is not possible, all **key players** should be given the opportunity to comment on the plan. If everybody agrees on the **outline** for each publication this will greatly reduce the risk of differences in interpretation scuppering the schedule.

Many contracts allow sponsors the right to delay a publication, usually to protect intellectual property (e.g. if a patent is being filed). Many sponsors also expect to be given the opportunity to review a publication before it is submitted. When planning a publication schedule you need to build this time (often 30 days, but sometimes 60 or even 90) into the plan. When planning to submit an abstract it is especially important to allow time for review by colleagues, institutional bosses and the sponsor.

As an individual contributor to a study, if you disagree strongly with the way in which the results are presented or interpreted your only weapons are your power of persuasion and reasoned argument. If agreement cannot be reached, you can withdraw your name from the list of authors, but you cannot veto a publication.

■ Vicious reviewers

A review of a paper should never contain disparaging remarks about the authors and should, in an ideal world, be courteous even if it is damning. If you receive a discourteous review you might mention this in your response to the journal but, especially if the reviewer recommends rejection, be careful not to sound peevish yourself and be sure to distinguish between the style and the substance.

See **zealots** for more discussion about consistently harsh reviewers. If you feel you have been the victim of an unduly harsh review, it may be worth appealing, but it is often best to try another journal.

W

■ WAME; *see* World Association of Medical Editors

■ Web publication / institutional websites

Most journals regard posting on a personal or institutional website to be equivalent to publication and you should therefore avoid this before your paper has been published. However, some journals, including some that otherwise limit access to subscribers only, now actively encourage such posting after publication. Before posting (either before or after publication) you should therefore check with the journal.

Journals that operate an **Open Access** policy generally permit authors to post their own material, or to include a link to the journal website from their own. **BioMed Central** has recently launched Open Repository, a commercial service to help institutions administer publication archives. *See* www.biomedcentral.com for details.

Perhaps surprisingly, most journals do not consider a 'webcast' from a meeting to constitute prior publication.[1]

1 Kassirer JP (1999) Posting presentations at medical meetings on the internet. *NEJM*. **340**: 803.

■ Withdrawal

If you discover a serious problem with your work before publication, contact the journal or conference immediately and ask to withdraw it. Despite everybody's best efforts and expertise, mistakes do happen, and most editors will appreciate your honesty.

However, abstracts and papers should not be withdrawn simply because a company's policies or priorities have changed. Some conferences accept **placeholder abstracts** which describe the design of a study but not the results. It is not good practice to withdraw these if results turn out unfavourably to your product or theory. Companies and researchers should commit to publishing all their studies, otherwise they will be contributing to **publication bias**. However, if you submit an abstract in good faith and then do not have any meaningful results to present by the time of the meeting, for example because of delays in recruitment, withdrawal may be acceptable.

If a journal discovers that it has published a flawed or misleading paper (either because of a genuine error or because of scientific misconduct) it may retract the paper. The notice of retraction should appear in indexing systems that cover the journal. Although, in complex studies, contributors may take responsibility for only part of the research, all authors (or contributors) will be affected by such a retraction, so think hard before putting your name on a paper if you have any doubts about it. Similarly, it is not usually possible to withdraw your name from a paper once it has been published – although, if serious problems come to light after publication the journal might allow you to publish a letter or statement outlining your concerns.

■ World Association of Medical Editors (WAME – pronounced 'whammy')

This is the newest of the associations for medical editors, founded in 1995. Unlike the **Council of Science Editors (CSE)** and **European Association of Science Editors (EASE)** it is a virtual organisation, relying on electronic communication rather than meetings. Whereas CSE is predominantly North American and EASE is largely European, WAME is more global, with members in over 90 countries. WAME has developed a number of policy statements, which can be found at www.wame.org

Members can also take part in an electronic discussion forum.

WAME has an Ethics Committee, which considers anonymised cases submitted by members and aims to provide expert opinion. This function is similar to that of the **Committee on Publication Ethics (COPE)**, although it is more international and does not involve any face-to-face meetings.

■ World Medical Association (WMA)

Best known for issuing the Declaration of Helsinki, which sets out doctors' ethical responsibilities when doing research. The latest version (issued in 2008) states 'Negative and inconclusive as well as positive results should be published' and 'Authors have a duty to make publicly available the results of their research on human subjects'.

For more details go to www.wma.net

Not to be confused with WAME (the **World Association of Medical Editors**).

■ Writing

If you started reading this book from 'A' and have reached 'W' expecting information about how to write scientific articles, prepare to be dismayed. Developing skill in writing will undoubtedly increase your chances of acceptance, but this is a book about publication strategy, and many fine books on writing have already been published. Sorry to disappoint you, but I recommend you go out and buy:

Albert T (2000) *Winning the Publications Game* (2e). Radcliffe Medical Press, Oxford.

Albert T (2000) *The A–Z of Medical Writing*. BMJ Books, London.

Fraser J (1997) *How to Publish in Biomedicine: 500 tips for success*. Radcliffe Medical Press, Oxford.

Goodman N and Edwards M (1997) *Medical Writing: a prescription for clarity* (2e). Cambridge University Press, Cambridge.

Hall G (ed.) (1998) *How to Write a Paper* (2e). BMJ Books, London.

Lang TA (2009) *How to Write, Publish and Present in the Health Sciences: A guide for physicians and laboratory researchers.* American College of Physicians, Philadelphia.

Strunk W and White EB (1979) *The Elements of Style* (3e). Allyn & Bacon, Massachusetts. Also available at www.bartleby.com/141/

■ Writing group

If one considers the first criterion for **authorship** set out in the **Uniform Requirements** (i.e. involvement in study design, or data analysis and interpretation, or data acquisition) it quickly becomes apparent that, in all but the smallest clinical trials, more people could potentially qualify as authors than can practically be included.

However, the recommendations made by the **International Committee of Medical Journal Editors (ICMJE)** go on to say that authors must also be involved in preparing or reviewing the manuscript. The distinction between potential authors and actual ones therefore often depends on who is involved in developing the manuscript. It can therefore be helpful to designate a writing group at the start of a study.

If writing group members are identified early, study organisers can make sure that they have the opportunity to fulfil this role properly, e.g. by being given a chance to review and comment on the data and shape publications. Clear communication about how the writing group will function should also ensure that everybody has realistic expectations about who will be named as an author, and who is expected to do what.

There are no rules, and until now little published guidance, about the ideal size for writing groups. To some extent, this will depend on the scale of the trial and the number of people involved in study design and data interpretation. However, it is possible for a small coordinating group to be responsible for a trial involving many investigators (and therefore patients), so sheer numbers can be misleading. Similarly, a relatively small trial (in terms of patients) involving complex, multidisciplinary assessment, might merit a longer list of authors to ensure that all aspects are properly represented.

The ICMJE criteria also state that authors should be prepared to take public responsibility for at least some aspect of the research. This is a useful rule in deciding who qualifies to join the writing group. Hard work alone does not justify authorship, and unless someone could stand up in public and answer questions about the rationale behind the study design, or what the results really mean, then they probably do not qualify as an author.

This means that the writing group may include members who do not qualify as authors – for example a professional medical writer, or an author's editor, brought in at a relatively late stage to coordinate the process of developing publications.

Anybody who made substantial contributions to the study design and interpretation of the data obviously qualifies for authorship and should automatically be included in the writing group. However, investigators who recruited large numbers of patients (i.e. were involved in acquiring the data) will only qualify if given the opportunity to be involved in the publication. The study organisers will therefore have to decide how many people to involve. This is sometimes decided by a simple (and therefore arbitrary) formula, such as inviting the top three recruiters, or the top recruiter from each country. So long as these people are given a chance to be actively involved in developing the manuscript they will fulfil authorship criteria but, to avoid unrealistic expectations and disappointment at the end of the study, it is important to set out the rules from the start.

In purely practical terms, so long as it includes members with sufficient expertise, the smaller the writing group, the faster the publication process. The more people who are involved in discussing, drafting and reviewing a manuscript, the longer it will take to finalise. However, the writing group needs to include sufficient people to do the work and to represent all aspects of the trial. Between three and six members is probably ideal for most studies. More than eight members (which may be necessary for large, complex trials) will inevitably slow down the process because more comments have to be taken into consideration and it will be slower to reach consensus. It is also harder to arrange face-to-face meetings for larger groups, and this may further delay the process (since a meeting is often the fastest and most efficient way to agree final wording, rather than endless rounds of e-mail comments or ear-bending telephone conferences, which also become unworkable with many participants).

However, keeping the group small should never be used as an excuse to exclude somebody who deserves **authorship**. The ICMJE guidelines clearly state that all those who qualify as authors should be included. The **Good Publication Practice (GPP)** guidelines also recommend that, whatever criteria are used to select authors, they should be applied consistently to external investigators and company employees in industry-sponsored studies. For more information about people who qualify as authors but are omitted, *see* **ghost author**(s).

So, to summarise:

- start to think about the composition of the writing group early in the study
- communicate this decision, or the rules that will be applied, to everybody involved with the study
- ensure that writing group members have the opportunity to make a real contribution to developing the publication
- do not exclude anybody from the group who meets the authorship criteria
- but, if possible, keep the group to a reasonable size (three to six members is ideal).

X

■ Xenophobia (geographical bias)

Geographical bias (which has to appear under its slightly exaggerated and rather pompous form because I could not think of anything else that began with 'X') definitely exists to some degree, and a good strategy therefore needs to take it into consideration. At its mildest form, it simply means that North American journals prefer to publish North American studies, and the same holds true for other regions. This may have more to do with journal editors knowing what will interest their readers than a bias or prejudice against studies performed elsewhere, but sometimes a bit of the latter probably creeps in.

The former editor of the *Norwegian Medical Journal*, Magne Nylenna, and colleagues demonstrated one type of xenophobia rather neatly.[1] They sent a poor quality paper to 180 Scandinavian reviewers, either in English or in their native language. Reviewers who received the English version gave it higher ratings, on average, than those who received it in their native tongue. This suggests a bias against non-English language papers, although the effect was not significant when reviewers were sent a higher quality paper.

Another study by Egger *et al*. found that reports published in German were less likely to have statistically significant findings than those published in English.[2] This observation may have several causes, including the fact that English language journals tend to have wider readerships and higher **impact factors**, which may lead authors to send their 'better' results to international journals and publish less interesting findings in national journals.

When planning a publication strategy, it is important to identify your **target audience** and its location. People tend to be more interested about things that happen close to home, and there may be important geographic differences in the incidence or course of a disease, or the way in which it is treated. Defining your target readership will help focus your discussion on the most relevant, and therefore interesting, aspects.

1 Nylenna M, Riis P and Karlsson Y (1994) Multiple blinded reviews of the same two manuscripts: effects of referee characteristics and publication language. *JAMA*. **272**: 149–51.

2 Egger M, Zellweger-Zahner T, Schneider M *et al*. (1997) Language bias in randomised controlled trials published in English and German. *The Lancet*. **350**: 326–9.

Y

■ Young reviewers

Selecting reviewers is perhaps the most important role of a journal editor. Since most journals do not pay their reviewers, editors usually try to create a large database to spread the load and ensure good coverage in all subjects. The biggest names in a field will probably be in high demand from several journals (and already busy people). Furthermore, one study has shown that younger reviewers (aged <40) tend to produce the best reviews.[1]

1 Black N, van Rooyen S, Godlee F *et al*. (1998) What makes a good reviewer and a good review for a general medical journal? *JAMA*. **280**: 231–3.

Z

■ Zealots and assassins

An A–Z needs an entry for 'Z', and, fortunately, a study of peer reviewers in *Radiology* provides the answer.[1] This journal asks reviewers to rate papers from one (accept) to nine (reject). Siegelman set out to discover if some reviewers recommended rejection much more or less often than others and he called these two extremes assassins and zealots. Reassuringly, nearly 90% of the *Radiology* reviewers were neither assassins nor zealots, but gave ratings within ±1.5 standard deviations of the mean; about 5% fell into each of the intermediate categories of 'pushovers' who generally recommended acceptance (and gave ratings 1.5 standard deviations below the mean) and 'demoters' who generally recommended rejection (and gave ratings 1.5 standard deviations above the mean). About 1% of reviewers fell into each of the extreme categories of assassins or zealots. Having identified the reviewers from their average scores, Siegelman examined submissions that had been reviewed by pairs of reviewers from different categories (e.g. by an assassin and a mainstream reviewer) and showed that the reviewers gave consistently different ratings, suggesting that the categories were valid and had not arisen because some reviewers had, by chance, received either high or low quality submissions.

Siegelman suggests that editors might reduce unfairness in the peer-review process by weeding out the assassins and zealots from reviewer databases. *Radiology* uses a computerised database that allows editors to monitor reviewers' average scores and thus select a balance of reviewers (or at least ensure that no paper is reviewed only by assassins or zealots).

While it is always tempting to consider any reviewer who recommends rejecting your submission a biased assassin, you need to remember that, in most cases, the reviewer is only advising the editor, not providing the final judgement. If you receive wildly divergent reviews it might be worth appealing the decision, although this can be time-consuming and it may be better to seek another journal. If you think your paper has been the victim of an assassin, you could use Siegelman's study to support your argument and ask whether the journal monitors its reviewers' performance.

1 Siegelman SS (1991) Assassins and zealots: variations in peer review. Special report. *Radiology*. **178**: 637–42.

APPENDIX 1

Further reading

Albert T (2000) *Winning the Publications Game* (2e). Radcliffe Medical Press, Oxford.

Albert T (2000) *The A–Z of Medical Writing*. BMJ Books, London.

American Medical Association (2007) *AMA Manual of Style. A guide for authors and editors* (10e). JAMA/Oxford University Press, New York.

Council of Science Editors (2006) *Scientific Style and Format: the CSE manual for authors, editors, and publishers* (7e). CSE/Rockefeller University Press, Reston, Virginia.

Fraser J (1997) *How to Publish in Biomedicine: 500 tips for success*. Radcliffe Medical Press, Oxford.

Godlee F and Jefferson T (2003) *Peer Review in Health Sciences* (2e). BMJ Books, London.

Goodman N and Edwards M (1997) *Medical Writing: a prescription for clarity* (2e). Cambridge University Press, Cambridge.

Hall GM (ed.) (2003) *How to Write a Paper* (3e). BMJ Books, London.

Huth EJ (1999) *Writing and Publishing in Medicine* (3e). Williams & Wilkins, Baltimore.

Hudson Jones A and McLellan F (2000) *Ethical Issues in Biomedical Publication*. The Johns Hopkins University Press, Baltimore.

Lang TA and Secic M (2006) *How to Report Statistics in Medicine. Annotated guidelines for authors, editors, and reviewers* (2e). American College of Physicians, Philadelphia.

Lang TA (2009) *How to Write, Publish, and Present in the Health Sciences: A guide for physicians and laboratory researchers*. American College of Physicians, Philadelphia.

Smith R (2006) *The Trouble with Medical Journals*. Royal Society of Medicine Press, London.

Strunk W and White EB (1979) *The Elements of Style* (3e). Allyn & Bacon, Massachusetts. *Also available at* www.bartleby.com/141/

Wager E, Godlee F and Jefferson T (2002) *How to Survive Peer Review*. BMJ Books, London.

APPENDIX 2

Organisations

(*See also* entries in A to Z section, listed under full names, for more details.)

- **AMWA** — **American Medical Writers Association** — www.amwa.org
- **COPE** — **Committee on Publication Ethics** — www.publicationethics.org
- **CSE** — **Council of Science Editors** — www.councilscienceeditors.org
- **EASE** — **European Association of Science Editors** — www.ease.org.uk
- **EMWA** — **European Medical Writers Association** — www.emwa.org
- **EQUATOR** — **EQUATOR Network (link to reporting guidelines)** — www.equator-network.org
- **ICMJE** — **International Committee of Medical Journal Editors** — www.icmje.org
- **ISMPP** — **International Society for Medical Publication Professionals** — www.ismpp.org
- **PhRMA** — **Pharmaceutical Research and Manufacturers of America** — www.phrma.org
- **TIPPA** — **The International Publication Planning Association** — www.publicationplanningassociation.org
- **WAME** — **World Association of Medical Editors** — www.wame.org
- **WMA** — **World Medical Association** — www.wma.net

APPENDIX 3

Guidelines

The following guidelines may be useful.

- CONSORT www.consort-statement.org

- Declaration of Helsinki www.wma.net/en/30publications/10policies/b3/index.html

- ICMJE Uniform Requirements www.icmje.org

- PhRMA Principles on Conduct of Clinical Trials and Communication of Trial Results www.phrma.org/clinical_trials

- STROBE www.strobe-statement.org

- The Equator Network www.equator-network.org has links to many reporting guidelines

■ EMWA (European Medical Writers Association) guidelines on the role of medical writers in developing peer-reviewed publications

© Librapharm Ltd (2005) Reprinted from Jacobs A and Wager E (2005) *Current Medical Research & Opinion*. **21**(2): 317–21. With kind permission.

■ The need for guidelines

Medical journal editors have expressed concern about the role of commercial sponsors in publishing research relating to their products and, in particular, about the

139

use of professional medical writers (who were not involved with the research) to develop publications. The issues about involving medical writers and the appropriate role of sponsors are separate but sometimes overlap. Although many guidelines already exist that cover the preparation of manuscripts for peer-reviewed publications, none specifically provides guidance to medical writers who prepare publications on behalf of named authors. The European Medical Writers Association (EMWA) has developed this document to provide guidance for medical writers and to outline the legitimate role of professional writers in developing publications.

■ Scope of the position statement and guidelines

These guidelines are intended for medical writers who develop papers for publication in biomedical journals or presentations for scientific conferences on behalf of named authors. The guidelines may also apply to authors' editors and others who perform substantive editing in preparing publications for submission.

They are intended to apply to any writers who work on peer-reviewed biomedical publications, regardless of who employs or hires them, i.e. they apply to writers who are directly employed by pharmaceutical companies or other sponsoring agencies, those working for contract research organisations and communication agencies, and those who are self-employed.

■ Development of the guidelines

The development of these guidelines has not followed a strict evidence-based approach, primarily because of a lack of published evidence on how medical writing practices affect outcomes. The guidelines were drafted following a Delphi consultation process among the members of EMWA's ghostwriting task force.* They were refined after consultation with journal editors, academic investigators, and medical writers working for pharmaceutical companies and communication agencies.

■ The question of authorship

Many journals have endorsed the Uniform Requirements of the International Committee of Medical Journal Editors (ICMJE)[1] (sometimes called the Vancouver Group). These include a section on authorship which may be helpful in determining who qualifies to be listed as an author. The Uniform Requirements state that named

---

*   The use of writers who have not participated in research to help the named authors to develop publications is sometimes referred to as 'ghostwriting'. This term implies that the writer is invisible because their work is not acknowledged or because it is purposely concealed. Similarly, the practice of omitting deserving individuals from authorship lists is sometimes termed 'ghost authorship'. We have avoided using these terms in these guidelines, partly because we believe that medical writers can have a legitimate role in developing papers, and we therefore want to avoid these slightly pejorative terms, and also because we feel they are misleading if the writer's contribution is properly acknowledged. However, the term was used for the EMWA taskforce.

authors should have made a substantial contribution to: (1) study conception and design, or data acquisition, or data analysis and interpretation; (2) drafting the article or revising it critically for important intellectual content; and (3) final approval of the version to be published. Authors must fulfil all three criteria and everyone who meets the criteria should be listed. Named authors should also be prepared to take public responsibility for at least one aspect of the research.

In most publications reporting clinical trials, a medical writer who has not been involved in study design, data analysis, or interpretation will not qualify to be listed as an author according to the Vancouver criteria. However, so long as they work closely with the named authors, there is no ethical reason why such writers should not prepare drafts of publications.

■ Financial interests and funding

The issues of involving professional writers and the interests of commercial sponsors often arise together, but should not be confused. EMWA encourages pharmaceutical companies to follow Good Publication Practice for Pharmaceutical Companies.[2] Research sponsors (whether they are commercial companies, charities, or public bodies) have a legitimate interest in the publication of the research they fund. Medical writers employed or hired by sponsoring companies may be involved in developing publications; their contribution and relationship to the sponsor should be acknowledged alongside other relevant acknowledgements about the funding and organisation of the research.

■ Authorship status of medical writers

Medical writers should not agree to be listed as authors on publications if they do not fulfil the authorship criteria of the target journal. To qualify as an author, according to the Vancouver criteria, the writer would need to have made a substantial contribution to the analysis or interpretation of the data and feel able to take public responsibility for the research. In practice, this means that professional writers are unlikely to be named as authors on primary research publications. However, they may qualify for authorship of review articles, for example if they have conducted an extensive literature search. It is important to note that by agreeing to be listed as an author, the medical writer takes public responsibility for the research.

Although the Vancouver criteria have been widely adopted, some journals supplement the traditional author by-line with a contributor list indicating each individual's contribution to the research and the publication. In such cases, it might be appropriate to list a medical writer who had prepared a first draft or made some other significant contribution to the publication. Any specific requirements of the journal in this respect should be followed.

■ Relationship between medical writers and named authors

Medical writers and study sponsors must recognise that the named authors are responsible for all stages of the publication. They should therefore ensure that authors are involved at the earliest possible stage, ideally when an outline is drawn up, or the key points of the publication (or presentation) are discussed. In the case of studies involving many investigators, writers should encourage sponsoring companies to form a writing group or identify the named authors at an early stage and involve them in the process of developing the publication or presentation in collaboration with the writer.

While it is understandable that sponsoring organisations will want to contribute to or comment on a publication, this should not prevent the involvement of authors at the early stages. It is unethical to invite investigators to be authors if they have seen only a pre-final version of a paper. Writers should therefore request that sponsors involve authors at an early stage in publication planning and should resist attempts to do detailed work on a publication before the authors have been confirmed and the content of the proposed publication discussed with them.

Medical writers should discuss and agree the content of a publication or presentation with the named author(s) before preparing a detailed draft. Getting the named author(s) to approve a publication outline and key messages is usually the best way to achieve this.

The medical writer is a facilitator in developing the manuscript, but the named author(s) must take responsibility for the content. If disagreements arise over the content of the paper, the named author(s) must always have the final say. If disagreements arise between authors they should be resolved by discussion – all authors must see and approve the submitted version and any subsequent revisions. Many journals now require confirmation that the submitted manuscript has been approved by all authors.

To qualify as authors, investigators (or others involved with a trial such as statisticians) need to have an opportunity to make a substantial contribution to the publication. This will usually involve commenting on an outline, or discussing key points before a first draft is prepared, then having sufficient time to comment on draft versions, and will always involve review and approval of the final version. Medical writers are often well placed to ensure that this process is properly carried out, by advising on timetables for review and ensuring that named authors have the materials required to perform a proper review (e.g. data tables and background literature).

■ Acknowledgement of medical writers

The involvement of medical writers and their source of funding should be acknowledged. Identifying the writer, either as an author or contributor or in the acknowledgements section helps readers, reviewers, and journal editors to understand how the manuscript was developed, and recognises the writer's involvement.

Identifying the writer's funding source ensures transparency and makes readers aware of any potential conflicts of interest. Medical writers should therefore ensure that the relevant journal's or meeting's requirements for financial disclosure, or other statements of competing interest, are met.

If writers are not listed among the authors or contributors, it is important that their role be acknowledged explicitly. Vague acknowledgements of the medical writer's role, such as 'providing editorial assistance' should be avoided as they are open to a wide variety of interpretations. We suggest wording such as 'We thank Dr Jane Doe who provided medical writing services on behalf of XYZ Pharmaceuticals Ltd.'

Although EMWA encourages transparency about writers' involvement with publications, because it believes that this usually serves readers and reviewers best, it also acknowledges that writers retain the right to withdraw their names from publications in exceptional circumstances (just as researchers who qualify for authorship may sometimes withdraw their name from a paper if they disagree with the way in which the research is presented or interpreted). Such a situation might occur if the writer prepares an outline or initial draft which is so substantially altered or replaced by material from the named author that the writer no longer feels that acknowledgement is appropriate.

■ Access to data

Some confusion has arisen over the specifications in the Uniform Requirements[1] concerning access to the data. It is not usually necessary or desirable for authors to have access to individual patient data listings, as results become meaningful only after the raw data have been analysed, and tables and graphs produced. This analysis should usually be done by a statistician rather than by a clinician. However, there will be occasions where access to anonymised individual patient data is useful (for example when reporting details of serious adverse events), and in those cases medical writers should ensure that the data are made available both to themselves and to the named author(s).

Both the medical writer and the named author(s) must have access to the relevant study data, for example a clinical study report, or set of statistical tables, before starting work on the publication. In addition, the writer must have access to the study protocol in order to identify secondary endpoints and analyses. Authors should not be expected to comment on a publication if they have not had access to the underlying data.

■ Writers' professional and ethical responsibilities

All medical writers, whether they are directly employed by a sponsoring body, or work for an agency, or as a freelancer hired by the sponsor, should endeavour to ensure that publications are produced in a responsible and ethical manner and that relevant guidelines are met.

Medical writers should be aware of any guidelines that apply to the publication they are producing (e.g. the ICMJE Uniform Requirements,[1] CONSORT for randomised trials,[3] GPP for industry-sponsored research,[2] and individual journal and conference requirements). It is the writer's responsibility to advise customers, colleagues, and named authors if such guidelines are not being followed.

Medical writers should also advise customers and colleagues about the conventions of peer-reviewed publication. For example, they should encourage clear trial identification by including an ISRCTN[4] (International Standard Randomised Controlled Trial Number), protocol or trial registry number, and discourage redundant/duplicate and fragmented publications.

Medical writers must strive to ensure that the publications they develop are accurate and scientifically valid. However, the named authors must take final responsibility for the content of any publication appearing under their names.

Writers must be aware of the extent of their expertise on the subject on which they are writing, and should ask for guidance from the named author(s) for any parts of the paper that are beyond their own expertise.

Writers and authors should ensure that results are presented in a responsible and balanced fashion. This is particularly important when developing publications sponsored by a company with a financial interest in their content, e.g. when a publication is sponsored by the company that markets a product described in it. The writer and named authors should have access to all relevant information and should ensure that all such data, e.g. full safety data, are included in the publication rather than selectively reported. The writer should also ensure that conclusions are fully supported by the data, and that publications do not contain unjustified claims. Secondary publications and post-hoc analyses must be clearly identified as such. Medical writers should also draw attention to any limitations of the study in the discussion section.

When preparing review articles (whether systematic or non-systematic), writers should ensure that the search criteria are stated. Even in non-systematic reviews, all relevant major studies should be included, and not only those that support the key message of the review.

If a writer is aware of good quality evidence that contradicts a point being made in a review, or in the discussion section of a primary publication, the writer should attempt to ensure that this research is cited.

■ Implementation of these guidelines

This document is intended to provide a framework for professional medical writers in developing publications. We encourage companies who employ or hire medical writers to develop detailed procedures based on these guidelines, for example giving standard wording to be used in acknowledgements sections or contributor lists.

EMWA affirms that professional medical writers have a legitimate role in developing publications and their involvement should not be equated with sponsors' attempting to exert undue influence over publications. In fact, medical writers can raise the quality of publications by bringing to the process language and communication skills, expertise in presenting data, understanding of publication guidelines and conventions, or time which investigators may lack. This position is set out in the accompanying position statement.[5]

■ References

1 International Committee of Medical Journal Editors. Uniform Requirements for Manuscripts Submitted to Biomedical Journals. http://www.icmje.org

2 Good Publication Practice for Pharmaceutical Companies. http://www.gpp-guidelines.org

3 CONSORT statement. http://www.consort-statement.org

4 ISRCTN. http://www.controlled-trials.com

5 EMWA position statement on the role of medical writers in developing peer-reviewed publications. *CMRO*. 2005; **21**(2): 317–21.

■ Background reading to EMWA guidelines

Angell M. The pharmaceutical industry – to whom is it accountable? *NEJM*. 2000; **342**: 1902–4.

Anon. Ghost with a chance in publishing undergrowth. *The Lancet*. 1993; **342**: 1498–9.

Anon. The tightening grip of big pharma. *The Lancet*. 2001; **357**: 1141.

Bodenheimer T. Uneasy alliance. Clinical investigators and the pharmaceutical industry. *NEJM*. 2000; **342**: 1539–44.

Davidoff F, DeAngelis CD, Drazen JM *et al*. Sponsorship, authorship, and accountability. *Annals of Internal Medicine*. 2001; **135**: 463–6 (also *The Lancet*. **358**: 854–6).

Horton R. Signing up for authorship. *The Lancet*. 1996; **347**: 780.

Horton R. The unmasked carnival of science. *The Lancet*. 1998; **351**: 688–9.

Huston P, Moher D. Redundancy, disaggregation, and the integrity of medical research. *The Lancet*. 1996; **347**: 1024–6.

Lagnado M. Haunted papers. *The Lancet*. 2002; **359**: 902.

Rennie, D. Conflicts of interest in the publication of science. *JAMA*. 1991; **266**: 266–7.

Rennie D, Flanagin A. Authorship! Authorship! Guests, ghosts, grafters and the two-sided coin. *JAMA*. 1994; **271**: 469–71.

Rennie D. When authorship fails. A proposal to make contributors accountable. *JAMA*. 1997; **278**: 579–85.

Rennie D. Thyroid storm. *JAMA*. 1997; **277**: 1238–43.

Rennie D, Flanagin A, Yank V. The contributions of authors. *JAMA*. 2000; **284**: 89–91.

Sharp D. A ghostly crew. *The Lancet*. 1998; **351**: 1076.

Smith R. Maintaining the integrity of the scientific record. *BMJ*. 2001; **323**: 588.

■ Good Publication Practice (GPP) guidelines for pharmaceutical companies

■ Aim

The aim of these guidelines is to ensure that publications are produced in a responsible and ethical manner. They are designed to be applied in conjunction with other guidelines such as those from the International Committee of Medical Journal Editors, the CONSORT group, and individual journals. In addition, they may be incorporated into the more detailed operating procedures of individual companies.

■ Scope

These guidelines are designed for use by pharmaceutical companies, other commercial organizations that sponsor clinical trials, and any companies or individuals who work on industry-sponsored publications (e.g., freelance writers, contract research organizations, and communications companies). For simplicity, the terms 'company' and 'employee' are used in these guidelines, but they should be taken to include all of these parties.

These guidelines cover publications in biomedical journals, including both traditional print and electronic journals, and oral/audiovisual presentations at scientific meetings. They cover peer-reviewed publications (such as original research articles, review articles, sponsored supplements, and abstracts) and non-peer-reviewed scientific communications (such as posters, lectures, book chapters, and conference proceedings). However, they do not cover promotional materials, which are regulated by specific national codes and legislation.

■ Publication standards

Companies should endeavour to publish the results from all of their clinical trials of marketed products. These publications should present the results of the research accurately, objectively, and in a balanced fashion. Anyone working on company publications should follow relevant external guidance such as the 'Uniform Requirements for Submission of Manuscripts to Biomedical Journals' issued by the International Committee of Medical Journal Editors (ICMJE)[1] and the CONSORT statement.[2] Additional guidelines relating to publications from company-sponsored research are also outlined.

■ Relationship between the company and external investigators

The contractual relationship between companies and external investigators or consultants should be set out in a written agreement. This should cover publication policies and ownership of data.

Companies should be responsible for coordinating the publication of multi-centre trials to ensure that they are reported in a responsible and coherent manner (i.e. results from data subsets should not be published in advance of or without clear reference to the primary paper and should not constitute redundant or prior publication). Therefore, companies should maintain the right to be informed of any plans for publication and to review any resulting manuscripts before they are submitted. Companies should not suppress or veto publications; however, it may be appropriate to delay publications to protect intellectual property.

All authors, external and internal, should have access to the statistical reports and tables supporting each publication. When differences about the presentation or interpretation of findings arise between company scientists and external investigators, both parties should work to find a mutually acceptable solution through honest scientific debate.

■ Premature publication

While it is acceptable to present abstracts, posters, or lectures at biomedical conferences before the full publication of results, care should be taken to avoid premature or inappropriate publication (e.g. through press releases). Most journals provide guidelines on what constitutes prior publication and impose embargoes on contact with the press before publication. These are also outlined in the ICMJE guidelines.[1] In the case of findings with major implications for public health or of great commercial sensitivity, it may be helpful to discuss with the journal editor the timing of publication and proposed approaches to the media.

■ Duplicate/redundant publication/multiple submissions

Most peer-reviewed journals will consider only papers that have not appeared or been accepted for publication in full elsewhere. Presentation at scientific meetings does not constitute full publication, so prior publication of abstracts or posters does not affect the consideration of full papers. These conditions are set out in journals' instructions to authors and the ICMJE guidelines,[1] which should be followed in all cases. Because journals do not accept duplicate publications and because they do not want to waste the time of their reviewers, it is not acceptable to submit a paper to more than one journal at a time.

Companies should avoid duplicate publication of the primary results of a study in peer-reviewed journals. Cases in which secondary publications might be acceptable include symposium proceedings, results of significant and scientifically sound alternative analyses, or grouping of data from more than one study. However, such publications should not precede the original publication, should reference the original publication, and should include a unique study identifier as described below. Full peer-reviewed publications should contain references to all previous presentations of the data (e.g. abstracts). Translations of papers into different languages are usually acceptable as long as the original source of the publication is clearly acknowledged.

Many major biomedical meetings discourage repeat presentations of findings that have previously been presented to substantial audiences; the guidelines for each individual meeting should be observed. However, there is no absolute rule against submitting several abstracts presenting the results of a single study to several conferences unless this breaches the guidelines of the individual meetings. Closed presentations to inform investigators of results should not jeopardize publication or wider presentation of results at public meetings.

■ Identification of studies

Identification of clinical trials by the use of a study, trial registry, or protocol number helps readers and those performing systematic reviews by making it clear when data from the same patients are being presented in different publications (e.g. in abstracts and then a full paper, or when interim or long-term follow-up findings or secondary analyses are presented). A unique study identifier should therefore be included in all publications.

■ Authorship

The ICMJE guidelines[1] are a good starting point for determining who qualifies to be an author, but they do not provide detailed guidance applicable to all situations. Furthermore, some journals have adopted a system of listing contributors rather than authors. Therefore, the individual requirements of different journals should be respected. Whatever criterion for listing is used, it should be applied in the same way to both external investigators and company employees. Companies should ensure that all authors fulfil the relevant criteria and that no authors who meet the criteria are omitted from the submitted manuscript. The order in which authors/contributors appear on a publication should be negotiated between all authors/contributors. It may be helpful for companies to outline authorship policies in the investigators' agreement.

■ Acknowledgments

The Acknowledgments section of a paper should list those people who made a significant contribution to the study but do not qualify as authors. It should also be used to acknowledge the study's funding and the company's involvement in the analysis of the data or preparation of the publication unless this is apparent from the list of contributors/authors.

■ The role of professional medical writers

The scientists, healthcare professionals, and statisticians who were involved with the design, conduct, and interpretation of a study (either as company employees or external investigators) should participate in the preparation of publications arising from the data. However, since these people may lack the time, expertise, or language skills to produce high-quality and timely manuscripts, companies may wish to employ professional medical writers to facilitate the publication process. The writer may provide publication expertise and assistance with writing, editing or preparing manuscripts, or collating comments from contributors. When a professional medical writer is involved with a publication, the following guidelines should be followed to ensure that the opinions of all authors are fully represented in the publication.

- The named author(s)/contributors must determine the content of the publication and retain responsibility for it.
- The medical writer should begin drafting the manuscript after consultation and discussion with the named author(s)/contributors. It is often helpful if the author(s)/contributors and the medical writer agree on an outline of the paper before detailed writing begins.
- The named author(s)/contributors should be given adequate time to comment on an early draft of the manuscript.
- The medical writer should remain in close and frequent contact with the author(s)/contributors throughout the development of the manuscript.
- The named author(s)/contributors should approve the final version of the manuscript before it is submitted.
- The lead author should be responsible for submitting the manuscript to the journal and acting as the primary contact for interactions with the journal editor.
- The contribution of the medical writer should be acknowledged.

The use of professional writers may be particularly helpful when companies publish the results from large, multicentre studies involving many contributors. The formation of a writing committee involving the medical writer may facilitate this process. While it is acceptable for professional writers or authors' editors to assist authors who have written editorials or opinion pieces (e.g. to improve the written style of authors whose first language is not English), it is not usually appropriate for them to prepare the first draft of such articles.

■ Responsibility for implementing the guidelines

Company employees who are involved with publications and people who are hired by companies to work in this area should be familiar with these guidelines. Companies should ensure that appropriate management structures are in place to implement the guidelines. Company procedures for the review of manuscripts should ensure that approval for submission is given in a timely manner. (Most companies have a procedure in place for medical/legal review or 'copy approval', and it may be helpful to append details of this here.)

■ References

1 Uniform requirements for manuscripts submitted to biomedical journals and separate statements from the International Committee of Medical Journal Editors. http://www.icmje.org
2 The CONSORT statement. http://www.consort-statement.org

■ Good Publication Practice for Communicating Company Sponsored Medical Research: the GPP2 guidelines

BMJ. 2009; **339**: b4330 doi: 10.1136/bmj.b4330. Reproduced by kind permission of the *BMJ*.

Chris Graf, Wendy P Battisti, Dan Bridges, Victoria Bruce-Winkler, Joanne M Conaty, John M Ellison, Elizabeth A Field, James A Gurr, Mary-Ellen Marx, Mina Patel, Carol Sanes-Miller, Yvonne E Yarker, for the International Society for Medical Publication Professionals

Authors and presenters are responsible for how medical research is interpreted and communicated. Often their work is the product of collaborations with other individuals (such as clinical investigators, biostatisticians, and professional medical writers) from around the world. Some or all of the people who contribute to this collaboration may be employees of research sponsors, contract research organisations, or medical communications agencies that may be funded by pharmaceutical, medical device, or biotechnology companies. The authors, collaborators, and organisations share responsibility for developing articles and presentations in a responsible and ethical manner.

The good publication practice (GPP2) guidelines presented here make recommendations that will help individuals and organisations maintain ethical practices and comply with current requirements when they contribute to the communication of medical research sponsored by companies. These guidelines apply to peer reviewed journal articles and presentations at scientific congresses.

■ Evolving standards

The conduct and communication of medical research, including that sponsored by companies, continues to be criticised.[1 5] Since 2003, when the original good publication practice guidelines were published,[6] the environment in which medical research is reported has evolved. The Declaration of Helsinki, updated in 2008, places accuracy and completeness among the primary ethical obligations of individuals communicating medical research, and suggests that "reports of research not in accordance with [its] principles should not be accepted for publication."[7] Information about clinical trials, including results, is being made accessible in new ways driven by regulations and guidelines from around the world.[8-15] Standards for the accurate publication and presentation of research have also evolved,[16] and new or updated codes of practice have been developed (table 1). The International Society for Medical Publication Professionals (www.ismpp.org) has been established and certifies the practice of individuals developing articles and presentations sponsored by companies. These guidelines were written in light of these developments.

■ Methods

The International Society for Medical Publication Professionals invited members with over 10 years of experience in biomedical publishing to develop these guidelines (figure). The 14 members named as contributors to this article responded to the invitation and formed the steering committee. The steering committee reviewed the original guidelines,[6] discussed items to be included in the revised guidelines (GPP2), and wrote the draft guidelines.

The steering committee recruited an international consultation panel by direct invitation and multiple open requests for volunteers. The draft guidelines were circulated to the 193 people who agreed to be part of the consultation panel for comment. The consultation process was conducted in confidence (table 2).

The 116 sets of comments submitted were blinded and collated, and members of the steering committee assessed and ranked them on:

- The frequency of comments received on a particular line number
- The critical or beneficial rating given by members of the consultation panel
- The steering committee member's interpretation of the importance of the comments.

Ranked comments submitted by steering committee members were combined into a composite rank, which was used to create the final guidelines.

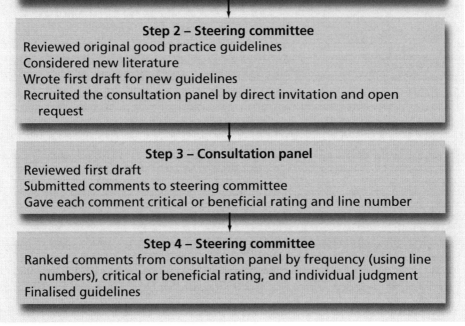

Step 1 – ISMPP
International Society for Medical Publication Professionals (ISMPP)
Recruited steering committee from ISMPP membership

Step 2 – Steering committee
Reviewed original good practice guidelines
Considered new literature
Wrote first draft for new guidelines
Recruited the consultation panel by direct invitation and open
    request

Step 3 – Consultation panel
Reviewed first draft
Submitted comments to steering committee
Gave each comment critical or beneficial rating and line number

Step 4 – Steering committee
Ranked comments from consultation panel by frequency (using line
    numbers), critical or beneficial rating, and individual judgment
Finalised guidelines

Methods used to write GPP2

■ Guidelines and recommendations
Roles and responsibilities
Written agreement
We recommend that companies describe obligations for good publication practice in written publication agreements with authors of articles or presentations and with members of writing groups or publication steering committees. We recommend that the written agreement confirms the sponsors' responsibilities to:

- Grant authors full access to study data
- Confirm the authors' freedom to make public or publish the study results
- Provide authors with copies of the sponsor's publication policy.

We recommend that the written agreement confirms the authors' responsibilities to:

- Plan and produce articles or presentations that are accurate and complete in a timely manner
- Avoid premature publication or release of study information

- Avoid duplicate publication
- Make decisions about practical issues concerning presentation and publication (for example, choice of congress or journal)
- Disclose potential conflicts of interest in all articles and presentations
- Identify funding sources in all articles and presentations
- Ensure authorship is attributed appropriately
- Acknowledge in all articles and presentations all significant contributions made by individuals and organisations
- Provide the sponsor with copies of publication policies from the authors' institutions

We recommend that the written agreement confirms the shared responsibilities of all contributors, including authors and sponsors, and that it:

- Confirms that sponsors will work with investigators, authors, and contributors to report and publish studies in a timely and responsible manner

- Defines the criteria that will be used to determine authorship for articles and presentations
- Confirms that the sponsor and the investigators will be informed about the publication process
- Provides protection to parties with intellectual property rights, and establishes a reasonable period before study results are made public for intellectual property rights to be protected
- Establishes the right of the sponsor to review, in a timely manner, articles and abstracts before they are submitted, and to share scientific comments with the authors
- Describes what, if any, support for the development of the article or presentation will be provided
- Establishes a process founded on honest scientific debate as the means to resolve scientific differences in interpretation of findings or study presentation
- Establishes that all articles and presentations will conform to good publication practice and other recognised standards (table 1)

Table 1: New or updated codes of practice since 2003

International Society for Medical Publication Professionals (www.ismpp.org)	Code of ethics
	Position statement: the role of the professional medical writer
Association of American Medical Colleges (www.aamc.org)	Report of task force on industry funding of medical education
American Medical Writers Association (www.amwa.org)	Code of ethics
	Position statement: the contribution of medical writers to scientific publications
Committee on Publication Ethics (http://publicationethics.org)	Multiple resources for editors

(continued)

Council of Science Editors (www.councilscienceeditors.org)	White paper on promoting integrity in scientific journal publications
Elsevier (www.elsevier.com/wps/find/editorshome.editors/Introduction)	Publishing ethics resource kit
European Medical Writers Association (www.emwa.org)	Guidelines on the role of medical writers in developing peer reviewed publications
EQUATOR Network (www.equator-network.org)	Reporting guidelines—for example, CONSORT, STROBE, QUOROM/PRISMA, STARD, MOOSE
Federation of American Societies for Experimental Biology (www.faseb.org)	Conflicts of interest in biomedical research—the FASEB guidelines
International Committee of Medical Journal Editors (www.icmje.org)	Uniform requirements for manuscripts submitted to biomedical journals: writing and editing for biomedical publication
Institute of Medicine (www.iom.edu/CMS/3740/47464/65721.aspx)	Conflict of interest in medical research, education, and practice
International Federation of Pharmaceutical Manufacturers and Associations (www.ifpma.org/fileadmin/pdfs/webnews/Revised_Joint_Industry_Position_26Nov08.pdf)	Joint position on the disclosure of clinical trial information via clinical trial registries and databases
International Society for Pharmacoeconomics and Outcomes Research (www.ispor.org/PEguidelines/index.asp)	Pharmacoeconomic guidelines around the world
Pharmaceutical Research and Manufacturers of America (www.phrma.org)	Principles on conduct of clinical trials and communication of clinical trial results
World Association of Medical Editors (www.wame.org/resources/policies)	WAME policy statements prepared by the editorial policy committee, including conflict of interest in peer reviewed medical journals
Wiley-Blackwell (www.wiley.com/bw/publicationethics)	Best practice guidelines on publication ethics: a publisher's perspective

Table 2: Consultation on first draft of GPP2

Place of work	No invited or volunteered	No agreed to comment	No who commented
Academic centre or university	10	4	4
Journal editor	11	8	7
Journal publisher	18	5	2
Medical communication agency, freelance medical writer	119*	83	52
Drug, medical device, or biotechnology company	109†	76‡	43
Professional organisation	21	17	8

* One email invitation was sent but not delivered.
† Two email invitations were sent but not delivered.
‡ One person was lost between invitation and opening of the consultation period.

We recommend that written agreements for articles and presentations from research studies are made at the earliest opportunity—for example, when the protocol is finalised. Written agreements for other articles and presentations (for example, meta-analyses, sub-analyses, review articles) should be made before the authors begin work.

Written agreements must respect the institutional policies of authors, investigators, and other contributors, as well as those of the sponsor. Individuals must not be asked to violate the policies of their institutions.

Access to data
Sponsors have a responsibility to share the data and the analyses with the investigators who participated in the study. Sponsors must provide authors and other contributors (for example, members of a publication steering committee or professional medical writers) with full access to study data and should do so before the manuscript writing process begins or before the first external presentation of the data. Information provided to the authors should include study protocols, statistical analysis plans, statistical reports, data tables, clinical study reports, and results intended for posting on clinical trial results websites. Sufficient time should be allowed for authors and contributors to review and interpret the data provided and to seek further information if they wish (for example, access to raw data tables or the study database).

Reimbursement
It may be appropriate for companies to reimburse reasonable out of pocket expenses (for example, travel expenses) incurred by contributors or pay for specialised services such as statistical analysis. Details of this reimbursement must be disclosed. We recommend that no honorariums are paid for authorship of peer reviewed articles or presentations.

Publication steering committee

It may be useful to form a publication steering committee of authors and contributors to oversee and produce articles and presentations from a research study. This committee should be a small working group of individuals; its composition may change over time, and it may include:

- Members of the study steering committee and the protocol development team
- Investigators and other individuals who have expertise in the area and who are willing to interpret the data and write or review articles and presentations
- Employees of, or contributors contracted by, the sponsor company who are involved in the study (for example, clinicians, statisticians, or professional medical writers)

Members of the publication steering committee may become authors, but membership of the committee does not automatically confer authorship. For any given study, we recommend that:

- The publication steering committee is formed early (for example, when the protocol is finalised or at the end of enrolment)
- All study investigators are informed of the committee's membership and responsibilities
- Authors and contributors agree to their roles in the development of an article or presentation before writing begins.

Authors

Recognised criteria should be used to determine which of the contributors to an article or presentation should be identified as authors.

We recommend using the criteria for authorship described in the International Committee of Medical Journal Editors (ICMJE) uniform requirements (box 1).[8] Guidance regarding authorship is also available from the World Association of Medical Editors[17] and the Council of Science Editors.[18] Criteria used to define authorship may vary among journals and congresses, and we recommend following individual journal and congress requirements when these differ from ICMJE criteria. ICMJE criteria allow assignment of authorship to individuals who have contributed to the analysis and interpretation of a study, but who may not have contributed to its conception and design. In these instances, or if authors differ from initial plans, particular care should be taken to attribute authorship and to acknowledge contributions appropriately.

We recommend that authorship criteria are applied consistently to all contributors to an article or presentation, including investigators, sponsor employees, and individuals contracted by the sponsor. All authors listed on an article or presentation must fulfil authorship criteria, and all those who fulfil the criteria must be listed as authors. All authors should agree on the order in which they appear in an article or presentation (if possible before writing begins) and should agree on any changes in authorship (for example, to ensure authorship reflects actual contributions made) before submission. Before writing begins one author (a lead author, who may also

---

Box 1: International Committee of Medical Journal Editors criteria for authorship[8]

Authors "should have participated sufficiently in the work to take public responsibility for relevant portions of the content" and should meet all three conditions below:

- Substantial contributions to conception and design, acquisition of data, or analysis and interpretation of data; and
- Drafting the article or revising it critically for important intellectual content; and
- Final approval of the version to be published

---

be guarantor) should take the lead for writing and managing each publication or presentation. One author (identified as guarantor) should take overall responsibility for the integrity of a study and its report.

Contributorship and acknowledgments

Contributorship and contributors
Interpretation of authorship criteria varies, and using a contributorship model to describe who did what helps to remove ambiguity.[8 19-21] We support this approach and recommend that clear, concise descriptions of the role of each contributor during preparation of the article or presentation (including but not limited to the authors) are made in an acknowledgment within the article or presentation.

Individual contributions to an article or presentation that should be acknowledged include study conception and design, conceiving the idea for an article, conducting or managing a study, collecting data, performing statistical analysis, interpreting data, analysing published literature, drafting a manuscript, critically reviewing a manuscript, and approving a manuscript. Permission should be obtained from each individual acknowledged.

Acknowledgments
We recommend that all articles and presentations include an acknowledgment, even if not requested by the journal or congress, to describe:

- Author contributions—for example: "A and B designed the study. C was the study statistician. A and C analysed and interpreted the study data. A reviewed the literature. A, B, and C critically reviewed the manuscript and approved the final version for submission. A accepts overall responsibility for the accuracy of the data, its analysis, and this report"
- Contributions to the article or presentation from people who are not listed as authors, including name and affiliation or employer—for example: "The authors would like to thank D, YZ Pharmaceuticals, for overall management of the trial and E, WX Medical Writing, for drafting the manuscript"

- The role of the sponsor in the study and its reporting, including how the sponsor was involved in the "study design; collection, analysis, and interpretation of data; writing the report; and the decision to submit the report for publication."[8] For example: "In collaboration with A and B, YZ Pharmaceuticals, designed the study, analysed, and interpreted the data, and edited the report. Data were recorded at participating clinical centres and maintained by YZ Pharmaceuticals. All authors had full access to the data. The authors had final responsibility for the decision to submit for publication"
- Funding sources, if any, for the research and for the article or presentation, such as for the work of a professional medical writer. For example: "The study was funded by YZ Pharmaceuticals, the manufacturer of drug F. Medical writing services from WX Medical Writing were funded by YZ Pharmaceuticals."

When journal or congress submission requirements do not allow inclusion of this information within the article or presentation, we recommend that it is included in a letter that accompanies the submission.

Professional medical writers

Professional medical writers work with authors to prepare abstracts, posters, slides, and manuscripts. They should ensure that authors control and direct writing and that disclosures of funding, potential conflicts of interest, and acknowledgment of contributions are made. They are required to have a good understanding of publication ethics and conventions, and ensure, in part through their collaborations with authors, that their work is scientifically appropriate.[21-23] Professional medical writers are not ghostwriters. The Association of American Medical Colleges states "transparent writing collaboration with attribution between academic and industry investigators, medical writers and/or technical experts is not ghostwriting."[24] This is echoed by the US Institute of Medicine.[25] We recommend that authors and professional medical writers working with authors use a published checklist to discourage ghostwriting.[26]

We recommend that particular care is taken to ensure appropriate acknowledgment of the contributions made by medical writers and to describe their funding. Companies funding the work of medical writers should ensure that writers follow good publication practice. We refer readers to guidelines from the European Medical Writers Association.[23]

Working with authors

Professional medical writers must be directed by the lead author from the earliest possible stage (for example, when the outline is written), and all authors must be aware of the medical writer's involvement. The medical writer should remain in frequent contact with the authors throughout development of the article or presentation. The authors must critically review and comment on the outline and drafts, approve the final version of the article or presentation before it is submitted to the journal or congress, approve changes made during the peer review process, and approve the final version before it is published or accepted for presentation. Authors may delegate to the medical writer (or to an assistant) the administrative tasks associated with submitting the article or presentation to a journal or congress.

As authors

Professional medical writers, depending on the contributions they make, may qualify for authorship. For example, if a medical writer contributed extensive literature searches and summarised the literature discovered, and by doing so helped define the scope of a review article, and if he or she is willing to "take public responsibility for relevant portions of the content"[8] then he or she may be in a position to meet the remaining ICMJE criteria for authorship.

Conflicts of interest

We recommend that authors disclose financial relationships (for example, any financial relationships or obligation to the research sponsor or other companies, including contractual relations or consultancy fees for scientific, government, or legal services, or equity in the company) and non-financial relationships (for example, personal relationships, including those of immediate family members, and participation in litigation) that could inappropriately influence or seem to influence professional judgment. We recommend that these disclosures are made in all articles submitted for publication in peer reviewed journals, as well as in abstracts and posters submitted to congresses at the time of submission, if space requirements allow, and that they are included in oral presentations and posters at the time of presentation, regardless of whether disclosure is requested by the journal or congress.

For example: "A is a member of a speakers' bureau, has been a consultant for, and has received research grants from YZ Pharmaceuticals. C is an employee of YZ Pharmaceuticals. B has stated that she has no conflicts of interest."

There is no universal standard applied by journals and congresses for disclosure of potential conflicts of interest. Until discussions about how to address conflicts of interest are resolved,[25 27-29] we recommend authors favour greater, rather than lesser, disclosure.

Recommendations for specific types of articles and presentations

Primary and secondary publications

A primary article is the first full report of a study. We recommend that all articles and presentations include statements to indicate whether they are the primary article or first presentation from a study, including for randomised clinical trials; epidemiological, observational, and descriptive studies; non-clinical outcomes research studies; and health economics studies.

Authors preparing secondary articles and presentations (including those that describe exploratory secondary analyses, national or single centre data taken from international or multicentre studies, and alternative analyses or pooled analyses of already published data) must avoid duplicate publication. All post-hoc and exploratory analyses must be clearly identified as such.

Authorship of secondary articles and presentations may differ from that of primary articles and presentations from the same study, depending on, for example, the topic of the article or presentation. We recommend that one or more authors of the primary article from a study contribute to the secondary articles and presentations from the same study.

Duplicate publication

We recommend that the same study results are not published in more than one peer reviewed journal article unless:

- The results are substantially re-analysed, re-interpreted for a different audience, or translated into a different language; and
- The primary publication is clearly acknowledged and cited; and
- The article is clearly presented as an analysis derived from the previously published primary results or is a translation, is not presented as reporting the primary results, and respects copyright law.

Presentations

Congress guidelines should be followed for presentations that describe study results that have been presented at an earlier congress. We recommend that, at the time of submission, authors disclose whether the same results will have already been presented at the time of the congress. With approval from the authors of the primary article, research submitted for presentation at national or local meetings may include authors who do not appear on the primary article (for example, to enable accurate presentation in the appropriate language).

Review articles

We recommend that review articles are comprehensive and that the methods for searching, selecting, and summarising information are clearly stated. We recommend that discussions in review articles founded principally on opinion are clearly identified as such. We also recommend that care is taken to ensure appropriate description of contributions from professional medical writers and other contributors, particularly when they may have contributed to the design of a review article or when they may have suggested the idea for the article. We refer readers to the *BMJ*'s "Who prompted this submission?" guidance (box 2).[20]

Box 2 | *BMJ*'s "Who prompted this submission?" questions[20]

We may ask authors submitting or offering unsolicited articles, particularly reviews and editorials covering topics with related commercial interests, several questions before proceeding. Even if the answers to all of these questions were "yes," we wouldn't necessarily reject the proposal or article. We appreciate that companies can commission some excellent evidence based work and that professional writers can present that evidence in a particularly readable and clear way that benefits readers and learners. We would, however, expect such companies' and writers' contributions to be mentioned in the article. And we would want to know that the *BMJ* article did not overlap by more than 15%

---

with any similar publications or submissions written by the same authors elsewhere. Here are the questions:

- Has anyone (particularly a company or public relations agency) prompted or paid you to write this article?
- Would/did a professional writer contribute to the article, and to what extent?
- Would the *BMJ* article be original, or would it be similar to articles submitted or published elsewhere?

Reporting standards

We recommend that authors follow established reporting standards such as CONSORT, CONSORT for Abstracts, STROBE, PRISMA, MOOSE, and STARD.[16] We offer the following brief recommendations:

- Articles and presentations should be complete, balanced, and clear
- Reference to the unique trial identifier should be included in all articles and presentations that report research from applicable clinical trials
- Interpretation of results should be unbiased, based on findings, and relevant to the audience
- Discussion of results should be unbiased, placed in the context of other relevant literature, and the evidence cited should be balanced
- Limitations of the study design and methodology should be described
- Studies with related findings should be cited, especially when previous results conflict with the results being reported.

WHAT'S NEW?

GPP2 updates earlier good publication practice guidelines.[6]

New elements include:

- An extensive consultation process was used to write the guidelines
- Authorship guidance recommends assignment of a lead author and guarantor
- Contributorship guidance recommends describing the role of the sponsor
- Recommendations about reimbursement
- Recommendations for specific types of articles and presentations
- Recommendations for publication planning and documentation

Updated elements include:

- Guidance on defining the roles of authors, sponsors, and other contributors
- Guidance on establishing a publication steering committee
- Confirmation of the role of professional medical writers

Planning, registering, posting, and documenting

Publication planning

Publication plans can help study sponsors ensure that clinical trial results are communicated by presentation or publication to the scientific and medical community in an effective and timely manner. They can also enable sponsors to identify the timelines and resources necessary to meet their obligations for reporting and publishing clinical trial results. Authors retain responsibility for decisions about articles and presentations from individual studies, which may be described in a publication plan.

A publication plan should support authors and publication steering committees (if they exist) in their efforts to ensure appropriate, efficient, and complete communication of results by:

- Identifying submission deadlines for relevant congresses and determining which studies are appropriate to present and might have data available in time
- Identifying areas for new publications (for example, subgroup analyses, topics for pooled data analyses, post-hoc analyses, systematic reviews) and the resources required for them, such as statistical analyses
- Avoiding premature release of results
- Avoiding duplicate publication.

Before publication

Research sponsors must register and post all applicable clinical trials according to the definitions and timelines required of them by relevant legislation and guidelines.[8-15] Posting clinical trial results according to the US Food and Drug Administration Amendment Act of 2007[10] and the *Joint Position on the Disclosure of Clinical Trial Information*,[11] whether before or after submission to a peer reviewed journal, should not preclude consideration for publication.[8]

Authors may present clinical study results at congresses before publication in a peer reviewed journal. Authors and other parties with access to study results should avoid further and more detailed public reporting before publication in a peer reviewed journal, unless the circumstances are exceptional.

Authors should not submit their work for consideration by more than one peer reviewed journal at any one time. All parties should respect embargoes set by journals, congresses, and other media. For example, authors should follow journal instructions when articles are "in press" or published online ahead of print.

Documentation

We recommend that companies, and the organisations or individuals working for them, document how publications are initiated and developed. We recommend that companies implement policies detailing the types of documentation to be retained, including:

- Agreements to participate in the writing process (for example, signed and dated letter, email)
- Details of intellectual input, direction, and contributions, including comments on drafts (emails, notes from teleconferences) or drafts that contain revisions

- Main versions of the draft, to document how comments on previous versions were incorporated
- Workflow and timelines that were used to develop the document, including time taken to review and revise the document
- Approval from authors of the final version to be submitted
- Lists of participants other than authors who were allowed to review or comment on the document.

We recommend that this documentation is maintained for a period defined by the sponsor company's retention policy.

■ Checklists

Articles and presentations following good publication practice will show the characteristics described in table 3. Written agreements using good publication practice will cover, at a minimum, the items described in table 4.

Table 3: GPP2 checklist for articles and presentations

Characteristic	*Check*
Integrity	
Accurate, objective, balanced writing	
Full access to data for authors and contributors	
Absence of duplicative publications	
Honest attribution of authorship	
Completeness	
Clear description of research hypotheses	
Reporting the detail required to ensure unbiased presentation	
Complete and honest reference to related work	
Use of unique trial identifiers	
Discussion of limitations of study design and findings	
Making public or publishing results regardless of outcome	
Transparency	
Making clear sources of funding	
Disclosure of potential conflicts of interest	
Acknowledging individuals who have made significant contributions, including but not limited to those made by authors, and by description of these contributions	
Recognising the contributions of research sponsors	

(continued)

Characteristic	Check

Accountability

    Being accountable for the work and, in the case of authors and presenters, taking public responsibility for the work

    Assigning a guarantor

Responsibility

    Making public or publishing results in a timely manner

    Respecting intellectual property

Respecting the responsibilities of contributing individuals and organisations for good publication practice

Table 4: GPP2 checklist of basic requirements for written publication agreements

	Check
Does the agreement describe the roles and responsibilities of the sponsor, authors, and contributors?	
Confirmation of full access to data for authors and contributors	
Confirmation of authors' freedom to make public or publish the study results	
Confirmation of the intent to report or publish studies in a timely and responsible manner	
Definition of criteria that will be used to determine authorship	
Requirement that premature and duplicate publication are avoided	
Establishment of right of sponsor to review articles and presentations and responsibility to do so in a timely manner	
Establishment of process founded on honest scientific debate to resolve differences in study interpretation or presentation	
Requirement that intellectual property rights are respected	
Does the agreement confirm that all articles and presentations will conform to good publication practice and other recognised standards?	
Was the agreement established at the earliest opportunity (for example, when protocol was finalised)?	

■ Acknowledgements

The International Society for Medical Publication Professionals initiated the development of these guidelines. The opinions expressed here do not necessarily represent those of the authors' employers. We thank the consultation panel for their comments. We thank Elizabeth Wager, Sideview, for her work on the original guidelines[6] that GPP2 updates (some of the earlier guidance remains in these new guidelines) and for her willingness for ISMPP to sponsor the authors to write GPP2. We thank Sheema Sheikh at Excerpta Medica, Elsevier for compiling comments from the consultation.

Contributors: Jane Moore, Medtronic, and John Draper, Peloton Advantage, were members of the steering committee and contributed to discussions about the recommendations made in this document (JD in particular on managed care, pharmacoeconomic, and health outcomes). CG wrote the first and final draft; WPB wrote the draft sections on publication planning, documentation, and conflict of interest; DB, EAF, CSM, and MP contributed to outline, intermediate drafts, and revisions; VBW wrote the draft sections on authors, contributorship, acknowledgments, and medical writers; JMC the draft duplicate publication section, JME the draft review articles section, JAG the draft publication steering committee section, and YEY the draft access to data section. MEM compiled steering committee comments after the consultation, and contributed to outline, intermediate drafts, and revisions. All the authors contributed to the literature analysis and review before writing these guidelines. All the authors contributed to the outline and to the first and subsequent drafts, to interpretation of the comments gathered during the consultation phase, and reviewed the final draft. All the authors approve this document and CG is the guarantor.

■ References

1　Angell M. Industry-sponsored clinical research: a broken system. *JAMA* 2008; 300: 1069–71.

2　Ross JS, Hill KP, Egilman DS, Krumholz HM. Guest authorship and ghostwriting in publications related to rofecoxib: a case study of industry documents from rofecoxib litigation. *JAMA* 2008; 299: 1800–12.

3　Hill KP, Ross JS, Egilman DS, Krumholz HM. The ADVANTAGE seeding trial: a review of internal documents. *Ann Intern Med* 2008; 149: 251–8.

4　Titus SL, Wells JA, Rhoades LJ. Repairing research integrity. *Nature* 2008; 453: 980–2.

5　Woloshin S, Schwartz LM, Casella SL, Kennedy AT, Larson RJ. Press releases by academic medical centers: not so academic? *Ann Intern Med* 2009; 150: 613–8.

6　Wager E, Field EA, Grossman L. Good publication practice for pharmaceutical companies. *Curr Med Res Opin* 2003; 19: 149–54.

7　World Medical Association. *Declaration of Helsinki: ethical principles for medical research involving human subjects, 22 October 2008.* www.wma.net/en/30publications/10policies/b3/index.html.

8　International Committee of Medical Journal Editors. *Uniform requirements for manuscripts submitted to biomedical journals.* www.icmje.org.

9　World Health Organization. *International clinical trials registry platform (ICTRP).* www.who.int/ictrp/en/.

10　*Food and Drug Administration Amendments Act of 2007.* www.fda.gov/RegulatoryInformation/Legislation/FederalFoodDrugandCosmeticAct FDCAct/SignificantAmendmentstotheFDCAct/FoodandDrugAdministration AmendmentsActof2007/default.htm.

11　International Federation of Pharmaceutical Manufacturers and Associations,

European Federation of Pharmaceutical Industries and Associations, Japan Pharmaceutical Manufacturers Association, Pharmaceutical Research and Manufacturers of America. *Joint position on the disclosure of clinical trial information via clinical trial registries and databases.* http://clinicaltrials.ifpma.org/fileadmin/files/pdfs/EN/Revised_Joint_Industry_Position_Nov_2008.pdf.

12 Legisalud Argentina. *Créase el registro de ensayos clínicos en seres humanos.* http://test.e-legis-ar.msal.gov.ar/leisref/public/showAct.php?id=12916.

13 Sociedade Brasileira de Profissionais em Pesquisa Clínica. *Legislação Brasileira Secretaria De Vigilância Sanitária E Anvisa.* www.sbppc.org.br.

14 South African National Clinical Trial Register. www.sanctr.gov.za/Investigator-brnbspInformation/Registrationandregulation/tabid/194/Default.aspx.

15 European Commission. *List of fields contained in the 'EudraCT' clinical trials database to be made public, in accordance with article 57(2) of regulation (EC) No 726/2004 and its implementing guideline 2008/C168/02.* 2009. http://ec.europa.eu/enterprise/pharmaceuticals/eudralex/vol-10/2009_02_04_guideline.pdf.

16 EQUATOR Network. *Library for health research reporting.* www.equator-network.org/resource-centre/library-of-health-research-reporting.

17 World Association of Medical Editors. *Policy statements.* www.wame.org/resources/policies#authorship.

18 Council of Science Editors. *CSE task force on authorship. Draft white paper: solutions.* 1999. www.councilscienceeditors.org/services/atf_whitepaper.cfm#5.

19 Rennie D, Flanagin A, Yank V. The contributions of authors. *JAMA* 2000; 284: 89–91.

20 BMJ. *Submitting an article to the BMJ.* http://resources.bmj.com/bmj/authors/article-submission.

21 Norris R, Bowman A, Fagan JM, Gallagher ER, Geraci AB, Gertel A, *et al.* International Society for Medical Publication Professionals (ISMPP) position statement: the role of the professional medical writer. *Curr Med Res Opin* 2007; 23: 1837–40.

22 Hamilton CW, Royer MG; AMWA 2002 task force on the contributions of medical writers to scientific publications. AMWA position statement on the contributions of medical writers to scientific publications. *AMWA Journal* 2003; 18: 13–6.

23 Jacobs A, Wager E. EMWA guidelines on the role of medical writers in developing peer-reviewed publications. *Curr Med Res Opin* 2005; 21: 317–21.

24 Association of American Medical Colleges. *Industry funding of medical education. Report of an AAMC task force.* 2008. http://services.aamc.org/publications/showfile.cfm?file=version114.pdf&prd_id=232.

25 Lo B, Field MJ, Institute of Medicine. *Conflict of interest in medical research, education, and practice.* Washington, DC: National Academies Press, 2009.

26 Gøtzsche PC, Kassirer JP, Woolley KL, Wager E, Jacobs A, Gertel A, *et al.* What should be done to tackle ghostwriting in the medical literature? *PLoS Med* 2009; 6(2): e1000023.

27 Stossel TP. Has the hunt for conflicts of interest gone too far? Yes. *BMJ* 2008; 336: 476.

28 Lee K. Has the hunt for conflicts of interest gone too far? No. *BMJ* 2008; 336: 477.

29 Drazen JM, van der Weyden MB, Sahni P, Rosenberg J, Marusic A, Laine C, *et al.* Uniform format for disclosure of competing interests in ICMJE journals. *N Engl J Med* 2009; Oct 13 [Epub ahead of print].

Index

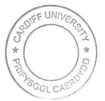